SOME

KIDS

LEFT

BEHIND

SOME

A Survivor's Fight for Health Care in the Wake of 9/11

KIDS

LILA NORDSTROM

LEFT

FOREWORDS BY CONGRESSMAN JERROLD NADLER AND CONGRESSWOMAN CAROLYN B. MALONEY

BEHIND

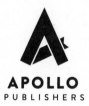

APOLLO
PUBLISHERS

CONTENTS

For my parents, who taught me how to rabble-rouse, and Kimberly Flynn, who advocated for me so that I could advocate for others.

AUTHOR'S NOTE

THE STORY TOLD HERE is based on my personal experience, and the events are written as remembered. It is not meant to be an exhaustive history of the downtown community's battles for care. Mine is just one of many 9/11 advocacy tales, so many of which began long before my own and helped create space for my work later on.

FOREWORD BY
CONGRESSMAN JERROLD NADLER

I think back upon my time at Stuyvesant High School with remarkable warmth. For so many young people, high school is a time of rich self-discovery, of youthful joy and exploration mixed with the growing maturity that arrives as you teeter on the edge of adulthood. I was no exception. It was at Stuyvesant that I pursued both politics and my interests in biology and rocketry, quickly discovering that I was far better at getting elected class president than I was at sending rockets to the moon. When I graduated in 1965, I knew immediately that I wanted to attend Columbia University so that I could stay involved in New York politics. My time at Stuyvesant had taught me what I wanted to do and who I wanted to be.

Stuyvesant was more than just a high school for me—it nurtured my passion for politics and provided me with the structure that made all the difference. But for kids like Lila Nordstrom, whose Stuyvesant experiences were instantly shattered when two planes crashed into the World Trade Center, that sense of security and exuberance was something they may never get back.

I was in Washington, DC, the morning of September 11, 2001. Upon learning the news of the attack, I immediately jumped on a train back to New York. It was a beautiful, blue-skied day, clear enough to see the burning wreckage in Lower Manhattan from the window of my train. When I think of that day, above all else, I think of the silence. The New York that greeted me when I stepped out of Penn Station was desolate and empty—no cars, no people, no vehicles, nothing. It was eerie. But I knew that forty blocks south of me, where Lila and her friends had fled from smoke and terror only hours prior, it was anything but silent.

As the pigeon flies, Stuyvesant High School and Ground Zero aren't much more than one thousand feet apart, if that. Just three blocks. It was close enough for Lila, only seventeen years old, to watch the planes fly into the Twin Towers from the window of her classroom. Close enough for her to see, with her own eyes, the tragedy of people jumping to their deaths rather than be consumed by the flames. At the same age as I was when I was practicing for my next debate team event, Lila was forced to witness these horrific sights and then hurriedly evacuate Stuyvesant into a maelstrom of dust, chaos, and fear, running through a city gripped by shock and confusion until she was out of breath and far from home.

On October 9, less than a month after the dust quite literally settled in Stuyvesant, Lila and her classmates were back at school. Parents and teachers had been assured by leaders like Christine Todd Whitman, then administrator of the Environmental Protection Agency (EPA), that the air was safe to breathe and the school was safe to attend. That was a lie. The school, which had been covered in dust by the collapsed towers and then used as a morgue in the days after the attack, had never been properly cleaned. As debris was removed from Ground Zero, open trucks full of asbestos-laden materials were parked directly below Stuyvesant's open windows as students sat inside.

It took over four years for the truth to come out: the air was not clean as promised but rather contaminated with asbestos and other hazardous materials; the school and its HVAC systems had never been properly cleaned; and the carpets, auditorium seats, and other soft surfaces students encountered every day still contained hazardous materials. What was not clear then sadly is now: the federal government lied. People like Lila—who trusted leaders like Whitman and Mayor Rudy Giuliani to tell them the truth—inhaled toxic air for years. Their bodies bear the consequences.

The federal government lied to people like Lila and put their lives at risk. In Congress, I did all I could to draw attention to this gross abuse of power while fighting for accountability and guarantees that the 9/11 survivor community would be protected and receive the help it needed. It was often a lonely effort. But Lila, wielding both a Stuyvesant education and the remarkable strength and conviction you find in those—especially the young—who are resolute in righting a wrong perpetrated upon them, made sure that I was never alone in this fight.

The first time I spoke with Lila about her activism was by accident. She was on the phone with my chief of staff when I, passing through, heard a mention of Stuyvesant. I was eager to talk to a Stuyvesant student about their experience, so I spent a few minutes asking Lila questions about the conditions at the school, the air-quality concerns she and her friends had faced, and how we could work best together to fix them. It was the beginning of a rich and long-standing relationship, one that only grew as Lila poured herself into the vital work of fighting for 9/11 survivors.

With an unflagging tenacity matched only by her remarkable capacity to stand up for others, Lila demonstrated political courage and savvy that belied her age. When reports emerged that the Environmental Protection Agency had lied to survivors, Lila thought not of herself and her heightened risk of illness after being forced to return to Stuyvesant. She thought instead of the countless classmates who were at risk, and she formed StuyHealth to advocate for them and share resources with the 9/11 survivor community at large. To this day, the group continues to be a hub of information and a valuable source of support for the survivor community.

Knowing full well that she and her classmates could fall ill with a 9/11-related disease at any moment, Lila worked tirelessly to ensure that the survivor community remained at the table and included in any legislation. Through her efforts, we ensured that survivors like Stuyvesant students, downtown residents, and office workers were covered in the 2010 James Zadroga 9/11 Health and Compensation Act and remained covered in the 2015 and 2019 reauthorizations. Lila refused to fight these battles from the sidelines, instead showing incredible poise and bravery as she shared her story before Congress in hearings, press conferences, and one-on-one meetings.

As Lila testified in June 2019 before the House Judiciary Committee, which I proudly chair, she said something that has stayed with me to this day. She hadn't even celebrated her twentieth Stuyvesant reunion yet, Lila explained, and already, five of her classmates had been diagnosed with lymphomas—and those were just the classmates whom she knew personally. Another student, a year younger than Lila, had recently passed away. These young people have just celebrated their thirtieth birthdays, and instead of celebrating, they are fighting cancer, mourning their lost friends, and struggling every day with the emotional and physical toll of what they survived on September 11, 2001. Lila demonstrated remarkable courage in carrying their stories to Congress.

Lila and her classmates never should have been plunged into adulthood so young with such violent abruptness; they never should have found themselves on a sunny Tuesday morning fleeing for their lives as the world fell down around them; they never should have had to find themselves thrown from worrying about AP tests to worrying about inhaling carcinogens on their way to math class. But little has given me as much hope for the future as watching how Lila handled such upheaval, her incredible resolve and earnest commitment to compassion revealed as she emerged as a voice for the voiceless. With Lila's commitment to justice, her dedication to serving as a champion for the vulnerable, and her capacity to deftly navigate the harsh, often vicious world of health care and politics, she has made a meaningful, lasting impact in the lives of not just her friends and fellow students but in the lives of tens of thousands of others affected by the attacks of September 11. I'm proud to have graduated from the same school as Lila Nordstrom.

FOREWORD BY
CONGRESSWOMAN CAROLYN B. MALONEY

On the morning of September 11, 2001, when our nation was under attack, seventeen-year-old Lila Nordstrom and her classmates fled for their lives.

Over the next few days and weeks, our government told 9/11 responders that the air at Ground Zero was safe to breathe and the downtown community that they could send their kids to school and go back to work.

And so, with her classmates, Lila walked back into the halls of Stuyvesant High School—with doubts in the back of her mind if it was really safe.

I can tell you from my time down near Ground Zero—that air did not feel or smell safe.

We know now, definitively, that those reassurances from the EPA and the US government put the lives of thousands of New Yorkers, including children, at terrible risk as they were exposed to deadly toxins that would end up making so many responders and survivors sick.

Now, as we approach twenty years since that fateful day, more responders and survivors will have died from Ground Zero–related health conditions than on September 11. The students of Stuyvesant High School, and the other schools in Lower Manhattan, have seen too many of their classmates fall ill and be taken far too young. I count this as one of our nation's greatest moral failures.

In the months and years since 2001, as we saw 9/11 responders start to get sick, and then those who worked in the area in the weeks and months after, and then the students—we knew what happened. And we had to fight with the Bush administration to get recognition of the size and scope of the problem and to take action to address it.

But, as Lila recounts, getting anything done in Washington is no easy feat—there are countless rejections and brush-offs, someone else always with a more urgent need. It's easy to get burned out and for advocates like Lila to turn instead to life on her college campus or her newfound freedom as a college graduate.

But instead, she along with the responder and survivor communities did the hard work to convince Congress that 9/11 illnesses were a real thing and needed and deserved a response from Washington. And so, we did all we could to raise the issue and make it impossible for Congress to ignore us.

Lila tells the story of the many efforts to get attention, and how hard that effort was.

For example, one year, for President George W. Bush's State of the Union address, I arranged to have members of Congress from across the country give their gallery guest passes to 9/11 responders and survivors including Lila, forcing the administration to acknowledge the problem. But, even confronted by these living examples—some of them sick and dying because of their exposure to the toxins at Ground Zero—the Bush administration still refused to acknowledge that it was the toxins in the air at and around Ground Zero that caused this suffering. The Bush administration left office without ever publicly recognizing the pain caused by those claims from the EPA.

And so, we continued the fight—which Lila helped to lead. Finally, in 2010, Congress passed and President Barack Obama signed into law the James Zadroga 9/11 Health and Compensation Act to create the World

Trade Center Health Program and reopen the September 11th Victim Compensation Fund. Naming this bill after James Zadroga, one of the first 9/11 responders to die from a 9/11-related illness, served as a reminder that we had failed to pass this bill before his passing, and we owed action to all those like him—who already were or would soon become sick—and their families.

It is thanks to advocates like Lila, who kept sharing their stories, that we were able to build enough support in Congress to pass the original bill in 2010 and then its reauthorizations in 2015 and 2019. I hope that with both the World Trade Center Health Program and September 11th Victim Compensation Fund now made effectively permanent and fully funded, we have offered responders, survivors, and their families some peace of mind that they will not need to worry about getting the health care or support they need and deserve.

These advocates ensured that when we said "Never Forget," it meant never forgetting their stories, their sacrifice, their pain—or the responsibility we had as a nation to be there for them as they were there for us. And for that, all I can say is thank you.

PREFACE

My senior yearbook photo was taken on September 10, 2001, and I rejected it immediately. It was only a couple of days into the school year, so I hadn't assembled the "look" I was hoping to be remembered by. Not that my ideal outfit was much of an improvement. It was just that when I looked at the picture that would identify me for posterity, I looked goofy. Young. Naive. Plus, having examined the photo with a self-conscious teenage eye, I was sure I looked fat. I didn't want to be remembered as young and fat. I wanted to be remembered as a mature, sophisticated, latent genius.

We weren't supposed to get our pictures taken twice unless something went drastically wrong on our first try. Acceptable grounds for a reshoot included a black eye or a broken nose, a hospital-worthy illness, or a morning-only natural disaster in Queens that kept residents of somewhere far away like Bayside from getting to school on time. Somebody behind me attempted to excuse themselves on the basis of their distress over a bad grade. At our school for overachieving obsessives, it was the only time in my entire high school career that somebody tried that defense and nobody sympathized. We, after all, were too busy trying to show our best angles.

Rumor had it that sneaking into another session was easy enough if you casually walked in with a different homeroom, never mentioned your previous picture, and dressed entirely differently, so I stealthily began preparations to get my picture done again the next day. That morning, I obsessed over my hair and wore more makeup than usual. I carefully picked out a new shirt. I even wore new shoes because, although they wouldn't be visible, it felt important I complete the outfit. My idea of fashionable, remember-me-for-posterity shoes? Silver Velcro sneakers that didn't offer much in the way of support but went with everything (or, more accurately, clashed equally with everything). There's no accounting for taste.

Despite my careful planning, there were no pictures taken on the eleventh. My high school, just three blocks from the World Trade Center, was evacuated before the photo company even arrived.

GOING TO HIGH SCHOOL in the age of Y2K was already weird. The end of my freshman year at Stuyvesant was punctuated by what was, until then, the most transformational mass tragedy of my lifetime: the shooting at Columbine High School that occurred in Littleton, Colorado, in April 1999. Before Dylan Klebold and Eric Harris went on that violent rampage through the halls of their high school,[1] the most traumatic thing that had ever brushed up against our consciousness in New York was when Mayor Rudy Giuliani tried to ban jaywalking.[2] We fretted about how we'd ever make it to school under that kind of tyranny, but we laughed about it. When Columbine happened, the media told us that life for students would be different and we believed them; still, the tragedy felt foreign. Maybe we had known cute acts of in-school rebellion like pasting pennies to the floor of the swimming pool or selling passes to a mythical cafeteria on the roof, but we didn't know anything about guns. How students could have had access to a veritable arsenal was beyond us. In New York City we all lived on top of each other. We didn't have room for secret arsenals.

In retrospect I can read visceral fear in the voices of the news coverage from that April night. That's because I now know what it's like to feel that afraid. What I felt at the time was a tamer kind of alarm at the realization that every student interviewed on CNN in the aftermath of the shooting knew the difference between the sound of semiautomatic and automatic gunfire. I hadn't even known there was a difference. I had never even seen a gun outside of a police holster.

Twenty years after Columbine, school shootings are a regular occurrence,[3] but it took me years to make the connection that the two experiences—Columbine's and ours on 9/11—would leave us in the same place. We would both be vulnerable, at the mercy of our health care system and its massive gaps. This broken system would compound our trauma by offering an inadequate response to our needs and inducing years of post-traumatic stress disorder, which, even without the environmental toxins and respiratory issues, would make anybody more susceptible to serious illness. We'd require constant advocacy, often from the traumatized kids themselves, the need for which would never seem to fully disappear, the money for which would never fully materialize.

Whether or not you're a free-market person, a single-payer health care person, a libertarian, a socialist, or something in between, it's hard to ignore the fact that, when we look at America's response to most mass tragedies, we're not exactly a nation of heroes. We're in the business of protracting the pain of victims in this country every day, and this fact is just as related to how we handle the aftermath of tragedy as it is to why we allow tragedy to occur in the first place. My story follows this pattern, but you could just as easily ask the kids of Flint, Michigan, about it. The kids of New Orleans. The kids of Houston. The kids of Puerto Rico. The kids of Parkland. The kids of COVID-era America.

The only way I could handle the protracted pain was to complain loudly and publicly about it, to approach politicians in the street, to knock on their office doors, to call for solutions in the press, but the obligation to engage in twenty years of advocacy is not a fair imposition to make on disaster victims. At some point the solutions need to be larger scale and proactive. Spending my twenties and thirties knocking on doors all over DC was a worthwhile endeavor, but it shouldn't have been an obligation.

WHEN I FINALLY GOT my school photo retaken, it was November. I had a sneaking suspicion that the smoke I could smell as I sat in front of the spent-looking photo drop might be dangerous, but I wasn't planning to do anything about it. The experience of 9/11 was still unfolding. Ground Zero dust was still swirling. For the reshoots, there was no strategy for sneaking into the line. My classmates and I all silently agreed that nobody would speak of the first session. We were all different people now anyway. My new "look" for the year was a gaze composed almost entirely of nervous expectancy. I don't remember what I wore.

In that moment I certainly couldn't conceive of what the future would hold; I couldn't conceive of a future that went beyond 2002. I didn't suspect that the very air I was breathing would take me on a journey that would end with another photo, this time in the Rayburn Room of the United States Capitol, posing with the Speaker of the House, Nancy Pelosi.

As I sat in front of the drop and tried to smile, I realized that I could hardly conceive of the past either. We had entered a new century, after all. Next to the scandals that had lost their sheen, alongside the impeachment and the contras and the Cold War, I shelved my former self. I left her there—that girl who never had to think to herself, *Is wearing new shoes a worthwhile risk to take if I might have to run for my life today?*

The answer, by the way, is always no. If there is anything that makes months of sheer terror worse, it's blisters.

CHAPTER 1

NEW SHOES

Some of us had experience evacuating Stuyvesant High School before September 2001. In the fall of 1998, during my first semester there, an interesting ritual developed. Every day at a different time the fire alarm would go off and the entire school would vacate the premises. We'd stand up from our desks, filter out of the emergency exits, and loiter for a while in various designated fire zones only to be called back to class soon after with no explanation. We did this for days without any idea why until a rumor began to circulate that an unnamed freshman—one of us—was setting a fire in a different school bathroom every day. The fire starter was clearly somebody who hadn't gotten the message, relayed repeatedly during our orientation, that if we didn't get straight As and act like obedient tiny robots for the next four years, our adult lives would be a destroyed, starting with our inevitable rejection from Harvard, followed by an unsatisfying marriage to a below-average person, and culminating in a life of abject poverty and drudgery. (I may be an unreliable source on this. I was exactly the kind of obedient robot that would have read a threat to lifelong happiness into any casual comment about good behavior.)

The ritual went on and on, and as the bathroom fires continued, the evacuations became cumbersome for an administration straining to find time for actual instruction. There were, at times, multiple fires in one day or inconveniently timed fires that ran across periods. Every fire caused at least thirty minutes of wasted time between the movements of thousands of students, the enthusiastic speculation about the culprit, and the time it took for the smell of smoke to clear. Eventually the administration decided to split the difference between safety and education and made a change. A few days into the thrill of perma-emergency, we were informed that instead of instinctively leaving upon hearing the shrill wail of the alarm, we should wait for an announcement telling us which specific floors were going to evacuate. Everybody else was theoretically to remain in class, lessons uninterrupted.

In practice, this system of waiting it out was just as distracting and wasted just as much time as a complete evacuation. At least once, the floors below and above me were given orders to leave while I was instructed to stay put. (For the record, there is no way to lean into a meaningful class discussion about *The Great Gatsby* while a fire alarm blares and smoke seeps into the room, even if you're assured that you aren't in danger.) Periodically, we would smell the familiar scent of bathroom smoke and wait patiently only to be given no instructions whatsoever.

After a while we understood that the fires weren't hazardous so much as annoying. The evacuations, which had created a frenzied atmosphere early on, began to feel more like very informal fire drills than actual emergencies. Anything becomes normal after a while. Soon many students were coming to school hoping to evacuate in that day's fire—it was a time to catch up with friends, confer about test answers, and, for some, a way to abandon class after attendance had already been taken. The overambitious half of the Stuyvesant student body continued to freak out about missing class time, but for most of us the later days of the fire era were actually fun. They felt formative—so formative that in my memory this period lasted for months. In reality it was probably over within a few weeks and dealt with via the swift expulsion of the culprit. Either way, it was a bonding experience for my high school class, a hazing ritual that gave us the authority and experience to feel at home in the notorious pressure cooker that is Stuyvesant. By the end we knew every escape hatch. Every door that led to the outside. Every back stairwell. The building felt like home.

Through the lens of my evacuation on the third day of my senior year, the fire era seems cute and quaint. A lot of people are surprised to hear that the prior classes had no such memory of school-wide evacuation—the day that Ramzi Yousef bombed the World Trade Center in 1993, killing six and injuring over a thousand, students at Stuyvesant stayed put and continued class.[4] The attack was an appropriate welcome to the neighborhood, nonetheless. Stuyvesant High School was founded in 1904 but was somehow never witness to a single terrorist attack until it outgrew its original home on East 15th Street and moved to its current building, a sleek new ten-story tower on Chambers Street, in 1992.[5] Since the move, there have been three major attacks within blocks of the school: the World Trade Center bombing of 1993, 9/11, and a 2017 Halloween truck rampage that ended right outside the school building, killing eight people and forcing the staff to answer questions about the previous terrorist incident.[6]

In 2001, however, thanks to the fire era, approximately eight hundred of us had a working knowledge of the school's complicated evacuation procedures, one probably rivaled only by whoever is in charge of designing those routes for the city. None of us got to put that knowledge to much use, though, because on the day the World Trade Center was attacked in 2001, there was not an orderly evacuation by floor or class as much as an open door to the West Side Highway and a vague instruction to run north and not turn back. What a waste of good training.

SEPTEMBER 11, 2001, was our third day of school. It was also an election day. When I woke up that morning the radio was, as usual, blasting the news so that it could be heard above the noise of horns and chatter bleeding in through our open windows. Yearbook photos were taking place all week and, having made plans to sneakily redo my shots, I spent extra time getting ready, trying to figure out what a person—any person—is supposed to do with hair. The unnecessary primping gave me time to soak in the latest about that day's Democratic mayoral primary. I wanted to be a good dinnertime pundit, especially since this was the last year that I wouldn't be old enough to vote, to actually be a part of the process. It felt especially cruel that I'd be turning eighteen just after the general election in November, missing the chance to vote for mayor by only days.

I love Election Day. I love voting. I love speculating about the outcome all day, then obsessively following election results at night. It's my version of sports. Election returns are all thrills and drama and heartbreak. The stakes are real and very present. The competitors, having spent months and sometimes years training for this very moment, are desperate to win.

I come by this electoral obsession honestly. Friends and relatives have joked that I was a "red diaper baby," a term that Cold War–era curmudgeons and radical-politics neophytes throw around to describe the children of the radical left. In reality, my family could be more accurately stationed on an outpost of the regular left. You could certainly get approving nods by mentioning socialism at our house, but when I was growing up, my parents were mostly ornery Democrats with union backgrounds whose marriage was largely premised on a shared love of discussing politics. My mother is a force of nature, and my father is the kind of guy who graduated early from every school he ever attended. He can handle having forces of nature in his life. All three of us prefer to shout our agreement over calmly acknowledging it. Of course, I learned the term "red diaper baby" when my parents let me and a school friend go on a trip to Cuba by ourselves at age sixteen, so do with that what you will.

The mayoral race of 2001 had been pretty exciting so far. New York City's public advocate, a showboating political veteran named Mark Green, was running for the Democratic nomination against Bronx borough president Fernando Ferrer, Speaker of the City Council Peter Vallone Jr., and City Comptroller Alan Hevesi.[7] It had been a dirty contest so far, complete with racialized caricatures coming out of Green's camp and the looming specter of billionaire Michael Bloomberg, a former Democrat running as a Republican, the monetary and political force to be reckoned with for whoever became the eventual Democratic candidate.[8] I'd been following with interest and disgust and horror and loving every moment of it.

I left for school with my head full of polling figures. School started at 8:00 a.m. with the dreaded "0 period," a time slot that was held exclusively for the unlucky and overly committed before school's official start at 8:45. If you planned your schedule right, you could make up a class during 0 period and leave at 2:15, but in reality, we all had to fill our college applications with extracurriculars or risk . . . I'm not sure what exactly, dying in the gutter? Missing 0 period or taking 0 period and ducking out early never happened. It was mostly an early wake-up obligation, and I've never been a morning person.

I am, however, an early person. I consistently feel a strong urge to leave my house thirty minutes before it's reasonable and, on the off chance that I am legitimately running late, the trains manage to run faster or traffic is light or everybody else arrives late and I still get there first. On September 11, I arrived at school at 7:30 a.m., as usual, and sank into a spot on the floor to wait. My chronic earliness means I spend a lot of time waiting around, and when that happens first thing in the morning I find myself calculating how many minutes of sleep I've lost out on in the process of being early. I'm still helpless to do anything about it. Because of this tendency I generally shy away from early morning obligations, but I'd agreed to the 8:00 a.m. class schedule because the subject was something I loved—architecture.

Stuyvesant was founded as a technical school, and all of us students had numerous shop requirements to fulfill as part of the curriculum. Some of our shop classes were famously challenging, but you could satisfy the requirement with less onerous ones like graphic design, which mostly involved easy art projects. Architecture was one of the most challenging of the shop offerings, but I'd always been interested in the subject, so after talking my way into honors drafting my sophomore year (the "honor" was based more on my gift of gab than my drafting skills), I'd decided to complete my final shop requirement by taking a double period of what was essentially advanced drafting with one of the department's most feared instructors.

Alphonse Scotti, a longtime teacher who'd seen retirement age come and go, hadn't much noticed me until my mother mentioned at parent-teacher night that I'd been carrying around graph paper pads and drawing floor plans for fun since I was a kid. By senior year he'd easily become one of my favorite teachers. I enjoyed his strict instruction and, while I was not a talented artist in most respects and was certainly no whiz at CAD (a computer-aided design software), I loved hand-drafting and I was decent enough at it. While I didn't end up pursuing architecture as a career, my handwriting is still a neat all-caps drafting font generally seen only on historic diagrams.

Mr. Scotti's classroom, along with the entire drafting department, sat on the tenth floor, an isolated outpost at the very top of the Stuyvesant building. Whereas the original Stuyvesant building on 15th Street stood out as a grand beaux arts monolith, the newer Battery Park City building blended in with the upscale brick-and-glass-clad condos going up around it. The school is nearly as well appointed as some of those condos, too. It houses a swimming pool, two gyms, a cafeteria overlooking the Hudson, escalators to help us scale the school's ten stories in the four minutes between classes, and a beautiful, though sometimes distracting, view of Lower Manhattan. In Mr. Scotti's class I sat with my back to the window, so it was my desk mate who, sitting at a drafting table overlooking the southern tip of the island out toward the Statue of Liberty, bore the brunt of the distraction.

On the morning of September 11, halfway through our lesson, Mr. Scotti was teaching us to draw straight lines or something of the sort.

Only three days into the school year, we weren't bored yet, but we were still teenagers in an early morning session who had been doing something incredibly repetitive for three quarters of an hour and knew we were only halfway through class.

Suddenly the sound of a major explosion shook me out of my line-drawing stupor. My desk mate's eyes went wide. The building shook violently, and when I turned around to look outside, a huge fireball had engulfed the North Tower of the World Trade Center. Mr. Scotti looked alarmed, but when he finally spoke it was to tell us to return to the lesson. He'd been at Stuyvesant in 1993 when a bomb had gone off in the basement of the World Trade Center. They hadn't evacuated the school then, so he assumed we'd stay put this time too.

Unsurprisingly, Mr. Scotti's "focus on the lines" approach didn't do much to calm the class. Isolated in the tenth-floor classroom, cut off from the escalators (the school's main transportation arteries only reached the ninth floor), I couldn't see how the rest of the school was reacting, but I suspected I should panic. Given our classroom's isolation, I was especially alarmed when I started hearing screaming in the hallways. As Mr. Scotti taught, attempting to keep the class calm, a student popped in from a room next door, where they had turned on the television, and announced that a plane had hit the World Trade Center.

That idea seemed absurd—absurd enough that I didn't really give it much thought as the fire burned. I watched as what looked like objects fell from the North Tower. I told myself that they were just construction materials—pieces of plaster, sheetrock, nails. I didn't worry that these objects seemed to move. The smoke made everything look like it was moving. For almost twenty years I've known that those falling shapes were people. In that moment, however, many of the important details weren't registering.

What did register were the sounds. Screams fled in from the street below, shouting surrounded us, and sirens blared from all directions. The first fifteen minutes of the disaster felt like hours, and during those "hours,"

I thought a lot about how every day on the way to school, as clouds moved passed the Twin Towers and made them look like they were migrating toward me, I would think to myself, *Those are too tall—they could fall on me.* When the first tower was hit, my first thought was, *I am scared*, but my second thought wasn't about the victims or how emergency services would possibly be able to respond to something this big or anything even remotely as generous. My second thought was, *I was right.*

Eventually a voice over the loudspeaker told us to stay put. A few minutes later, something with wings pierced the shadow of the fires. I assumed it was a curious, death-defying bird. It was a plane. We heard another huge explosion.

I've thought a lot about the fact that the second plane, which passed directly by my window, was the last plane in my life that I didn't pay attention to. It was the last time that I didn't track an aircraft's path until I could be sure it would make it out of view. Since 2001, I have lost hours of my life, little moments every day, to watching planes go by. Despite all that was going on, 9:02 a.m. on September 11, 2001, was the last minute of my life that was free of the obligation of noticing.

We felt the South Tower's explosion rattle the building, but our view of the impact was partially obscured by the ball of fire and smoke gushing out of the North Tower, so we didn't know for sure whether both buildings had been hit until a crew of roving hallway gossips confirmed it for us. My teacher continued with the lesson, more forcefully than before but with less authority, as we begged him to turn on the television. Eventually, over the PA system, the school administration's periodic admonitions to stay put started to sound more panicked and unsure. They would trail off on the intercom, discussion lingering in the background of whatever room they were in. It felt like the administration was getting contradictory instructions, which the school newspaper later confirmed was true.[9]

For nearly an hour we remained in a weird kind of stasis, waiting for instructions as we watched tens of thousands of people stream past the school on the sidewalk below, trudging uptown in their office wear. Our initial panic began to subside because the waiting game went on for so long that we had to begin the process of adjusting. My teacher continued with the lesson until it became clear that we weren't really in a class period anymore, just a never-ending waiting game.

As the minutes went by, the panic began to morph, like it had during the fire era. What began as stress turned, at various moments, into humor, into tears, into comradery. I experienced stretches of time as if I was on pause, too, waiting for somebody to push play and move us into a new phase of the disaster. In the waiting, the burning buildings became more familiar. Eventually they started to seem like a regular part of the downtown panorama. We hesitantly hoped we had reached the end of the surprises. Then, just before 10:00 a.m., the South Tower fell.

It felt like an earthquake. Our lights flickered. Sounds of panic echoed from every corner as people screamed out of their windows and on the street below. From where we sat, the North Tower's fire continued to partially obstruct our view, so it was initially hard to see the cause of the quickly expanding dust cloud roaring toward our windows. It was clear, however, that somebody had pushed play. We'd entered the next phase of the crisis. I watched below as the Applebee's across the street disappeared into a layer of thick, fast-moving dust.

Applebee's is a hallmark of the suburban experience, commonplace almost everywhere in the United States, but the chain restaurant was a rarity in New York City at the time. I'd been there once to attend a cross-country team dinner and was pleased to find out that it was, in fact, mediocre, quelling my fears about missing out on life somewhere else. On that day, without any context to comprehend the larger disaster unfolding, my mind oscillated between a slew of peculiar thoughts. As the South Tower crumbled and took out Applebee's, I thought about the fact that this was really the first and only time I'd seen Giuliani's Disneyfied New York (the incursion of chain dining being a prime symbol of "new" New York's corporate glory) defeated. I almost expected the Applebee's to behave like a New York City cockroach and refuse to disappear into the cloud, but it, like everything around us, vanished.

As the dust reached our windows, I started to feel the kind of subconscious anxiety I feel at my first whiff of cigarette smoke, the anxiety of being an asthmatic who is about to suffer. I was a sitting duck watching an asthma attack roll toward me. I confidently informed Mr. Scotti that I'd be going to the nurse's office—located more conveniently on a low floor near the north exit and away from the contaminated windows. I didn't ask, because I knew he'd say no—adults always say no when you want to escape a danger they aren't perceiving. I walked out without giving him a chance to comment.

I ran from the tenth floor to the third floor, television noise blaring from every doorway, lost and confused students crying in the hallways. As I made my way down, the PA system croaked on again and students were told to go to their homerooms to await further instruction. I had already passed my eighth-floor homeroom and had no intention of going back since it faced the same dusty windows. I did vaguely worry that I wouldn't be accounted for later, as if attendance in homeroom would be the only way for my family to identify my whereabouts, but being near an exit was my main priority. If I'd learned anything in the fire era, it was that fire drills start out orderly and get more chaotic the farther you are from the exit. I wanted to evacuate with the orderly group.

Stuyvesant has a program for disabled students housed in its building, and most of these students were in the nurse's office when I arrived. Students and their aides huddled around a radio, listening to screaming, largely uninformed reporting. The latest news was that seemingly hundreds of planes were still in the sky and every single one was headed for a New York City landmark. That, to us, meant that the plan we were discussing in the office, the gist of which was to walk north for as long as possible, could be compromised at any moment by another attack. It was the first time it occurred to me that Manhattan, which felt to me like the center of everything, is an actual island. It's not an island like Coney Island, in its "this was once an island before landfill was invented" way. It's surrounded by water. You can't just run off of an island.

When evacuation orders did come over the intercom, I'd like to say I helped usher the kids in their walkers and motorized wheelchairs out of the nurse's office, but what I actually did was bolt up without comment, run to the staircase across the hall, and scamper alone down the stairs.[10] I was operating on pure instinct. I wasn't even consciously aware of what was moving my feet. Our instructions were incredibly vague—just walk north. There was no designated spot to meet at later. Nowhere to aim for. We were simply told to get out of Lower Manhattan as quickly as possible and then figure it out. For those of us from the fire era, this evacuation was scary enough, but there were nearly eight hundred kids for whom this was their first week of school. Many had never even been to Manhattan alone before and lived hours away by trains that weren't running. A classmate who was interested in photography left the school a little early and took photos of students running uptown. The photos are striking because, though we were all young, some of the kids running uptown alone, panting, in tears, scared for their lives, still look like middle schoolers.

A few people made it outside before me, but the bulk of the student body was still inside as I stepped into a crowd of shell-shocked strangers walking between the West Side Highway and the Hudson River. In stepping outside, I immediately lost sight of anybody that I recognized, but I didn't have much time to think about it because as soon as my foot hit the pavement, a slow rumble began. There was no time to identify dangers and react to them one by one. Everybody around me took off in a sprint, assuming the sound came from a wave of thousands of people behind us, ready to trample. I ran too. Mid-sprint, I turned around just in time to see the antenna of the second tower plummet straight down, sending another wave of momentum into the dust cloud that had settled half a block behind me.

Asthmatics do not make for great sprinters, so I ran out of breath quickly. As I panted only a couple blocks north of where I'd started, I saw a familiar face and flagged her down. It was Anetta Luczak, a physical education teacher who'd taught my health class the year before.

Ms. Luczak and I didn't have much of a rapport before we ran into each other that day. At the time she seemed generally grown up, essentially adult, but years later I learned that she was only twenty-six and in her second year of teaching. She, like me, had no idea what she was doing. She took my arm and we began to walk uptown together, speculating about what else had been or would be hit. Cars had pulled over on the West Side Highway and were blasting the radio so those of us evacuating could hear the news, but the news was still a chaos of rattled voices declaring that every plane not currently on the ground was probably going to hit the Empire State Building or the Brooklyn Bridge or the George Washington Bridge or Times Square or . . . At a certain point all we could take away from the noise was an urgency to keep our wits about us.

We walked for a while by ourselves. While we walked, we discussed our options with a stoic practicality. From what we knew, they—the unnamed authority we kept hearing about on the news—were likely evacuating Manhattan. (This turned out to be false—they only evacuated Lower Manhattan, but the radio didn't know that yet.) That didn't leave us many options.

"Do you think we can walk to the George Washington Bridge? It's more than a hundred blocks away. Or was it already hit?"

Ms. Luczak shrugged. It was impossible to predict what was or wasn't going to be hit by a plane. "Could we get on a boat?" she asked.

We looked out at the water. Saw nothing headed in our direction. Ferry boats and water taxis were converging, but farther downtown.

"Plus, how would we get home from New Jersey if the bridges are hit?" I wondered aloud. Nothing sounds more threatening to a New Yorker than the prospect of getting stuck in New Jersey. We regrouped but quickly realized that there weren't many more alluring options.

Eyeing the water once more, Ms. Luczak finally said, "I think we might have to swim across the river."

My eyes widened. The water suddenly looked less like an escape hatch and more like a threatening abyss. I told her of a secret shame that many native New Yorkers can relate to. "I don't know how to swim."

Ms. Luczak didn't skip a beat. She, conveniently, taught swimming at Stuyvesant and told me, "I can swim you across."

Over the years, people have regularly second-guessed my evacuation decisions. Why didn't I get on a bus? (There were none.) Why didn't I go to a friend's house downtown? (I couldn't find any.) Why didn't I hop into a cab and joyride around the city? (No cash.) Why didn't I call my parents? (My phone didn't work.) Usually, however, Ms. Luczak's swimming comment is what makes those people the most upset. As if, even while caught in a wildly unrealistic situation in which the World Trade Center is falling down, a person should know that swimming across the Hudson River is absurd. As if she should have sucked it up for the sake of us kids and devised a practical, time-tested, well-considered game plan on the spot instead of suggesting the heroic, yet hysterical, swimming suggestion.

I doubt anybody who knows her has ever accused Anetta Luczak, a stoic Eastern European physical education teacher, of being hysterical, but I also think people's extreme reactions to her comment are an interesting window into how hard it is to comprehend what it's like on the ground in an unprecedented, extraordinary situation. Out of context, her offer to swim me to New Jersey sounds so ridiculous that it could be the punch line to a joke, but the offer wasn't really about swimming. She correctly intuited that I needed to be part of a team. Her offer to swim me to New Jersey was meant to be a sign that we were responsible for each other. It was the nicest and most comforting thing anybody said to me that day.

Despite the chaos of the evacuation, many of the teachers at Stuyvesant wound up shepherding a group of terrified teenagers to safety.[11] I've spoken to teachers over the course of the last twenty years who remember evacuating with kids whose names they didn't even learn. They traveled with these kids for hours, brought them home, met some of their parents, remember their faces. Some have asked whether those kids would remember them because of how confusing that day was and how haphazardly they wound up accumulating in these groups. I always assure teachers that their students do remember them—nobody forgets whom they evacuated with on September 11. For us, any adult taking control in that situation, even if that adult was only twenty-six and in their second year of teaching, was practicing an extraordinary kindness.

Like many teacher and student duos, Ms. Luczak and I eventually began to accumulate other students, some of whom had stopped and waited along the West Side Highway, searching for familiar faces, others who caught up to us as they walked uptown. Among them was a friend I'd been in homeroom with since freshman year, Laura. I should note that Laura remembers us being together inside the school as well, before getting separated as the second tower collapsed. Traumatic memories are notoriously unreliable, so I can't even speculate about which of us is right, but I know that Laura became the main protagonist in my evacuation story as soon as we connected (or reconnected) along the river. We'd been casual friends for a long time, but not the kind who spend time together outside of school. As we fled Lower Manhattan, however, she was suddenly the most important person in my life.

Stuyvesant draws students from all over the city, and most of our evacuee group was from the outer boroughs—an especially Brooklyn-heavy contingent—so as we trudged uptown, I was the first person faced with a choice to make about whether to go home or keep pushing farther away from the scene. My family lived in Chelsea, about three miles from the World Trade Center site, but I began worrying about my parents' house long before we hit 23rd Street, Chelsea's main east–west thoroughfare. Our house was far enough from Ground Zero, but what we lacked in proximity to the WTC we made up for in proximity to the Empire State Building.

That slightly smaller but heavier-seeming skyscraper was only a few blocks away from my apartment and was still being discussed on the radio as a likely target for attack. I knew my father, whose office was also in the area, was probably expecting me. Our cell phones weren't working—I'd seen the main cellular antenna downtown falling as the second tower collapsed—so I couldn't get in touch with him to find out what kind of condition the neighborhood was in. I decided to continue walking uptown. If they really were going to evacuate Manhattan, I wanted to get on my way. Laura offered that I could come home with her, and so her house in Queens, which I had never visited before and which contained her family whom I'd never met, became my destination.

Somebody eventually got word around 59th Street that the trains were running again. Ms. Luczak made sure Laura and I knew where we were headed, gave us big hugs, and split off with the kids going to Brooklyn. On our own, we turned right on 59th Street and headed across town toward the 59th Street Bridge.

At around this time, I made one of what had been many attempts to place a call on my cell phone, and it miraculously went through. My father answered, his voice unusually high-pitched. I was, by that point, so wrapped up in my present activities—in my urgent need to keep walking—that it caught me by surprise that my father had opinions about where I should go and what I should do. I told him I was headed toward Queens, and he told me that he had gone downtown looking for me, been worried sick, and that I should go home. I had already passed our house and, based on what I'd last heard on a random car radio, told him they were evacuating Manhattan. "I have to leave," I insisted. He hadn't heard about the island-wide evacuation, probably because it wasn't true.

My mother still complains that my dad should have instructed me to meet her at the school she taught at, which was on the east side not far from 59th Street. I'm glad he didn't think to do that. In fact, it only recently occurred to me that my dad, running downtown, and my mom, working at a school in Midtown and responsible for a bunch of small children, really had no context for what I'd just been through. They knew what had happened on a factual level—there had been an attack on the World Trade Center, the Twin Towers had collapsed—but they didn't know where I fit into that story. That's why they were so surprised that I didn't head home or to one of them, which, to their minds, was the same as heading to safety.

In my mind, there was nowhere in Manhattan that meant *safety*. The sounds of fighter jets soaring overhead had been sending our evacuee group into a panic. The unusual behavior of the crowd we trudged uptown with, along with the wild range of screams, cries, and absolute calm, heightened our alarm further. I felt a visceral need to get away. The danger wasn't sequestered downtown, it was everywhere—it lived in the panicked shouts and unknown threats still circulating between Downtown and Midtown. Our apartment was sandwiched between the two areas, but my parents were a bit removed from the excitement. They had room to be a little amazed by what was going on and to even think, *My daughter is down there—I should head* toward *the danger*. Everybody's definition of "safety" can only be based on what they know at the time.

This dissonance is an ongoing theme in my life. Watching the World Trade Center fall down from far away, whether live or on television, was different from watching it unfold downtown. People who were enveloped in the dust cloud's blanket of darkness probably feel the same disconnection to people like me who were never actually inside the dust cloud. To them, those of us who didn't breathe in the gray, opaque air did not experience the same emergency they did. We were removed from the action. When I watched footage of the towers falling later that day on the news, it looked like a sequence from an action movie. The experience of watching them fall on TV has nothing to do with the experience of watching them fall in person. They are two separate memories.

As I rushed uptown to get away from everything, my parents were reacting to a different terror—the one that came with knowing their child was in danger. They wanted me to be with them because then they'd know I was safe. I, meanwhile, had the suspicion that in order to feel safe myself, I needed to be in charge of my own actions and whereabouts and that I'd lose that ability as soon as my parents were back on the scene trying to take care of me. I knew from experience that they'd be less cautious than I wanted to be. It would take them too long to react to potential dangers, because nothing earth-shatteringly dangerous had happened to them that day. If we were ordered to leave Manhattan, they'd want to go get the car and some supplies and pack a little bit, and we'd get on the road just about the time that every other Chelsea resident dragged themselves outside against their will and organized their stuff and got behind the wheel.

I had different priorities. I wanted to be light on my feet and go to a place no terrorist would think to hit. Astoria, among its many positive qualities as a very pretty neighborhood with good Greek food, was also unlikely to be a terrorist target. To me, it didn't have the kind of symbolic value that warranted an attack, but it did have somebody's parents, and that seemed like a good deal. We continued on our way.

As Laura and I crossed 59th Street around noon on 9/11, people were eating leisurely lunches at sidewalk cafés, baking in the sun, and enjoying the wealth of people-watching available as evacuees migrated by. I remember one man in particular loosening his tie as if he were a television character pantomiming the universal signal for "businessman relaxing."

Most people begin their September 11 story with how nice the weather was. For some reason that's supposed to make the contrast of the day's eventual carnage and destruction seem more shocking; as if to say, in retrospect, we should have realized that it was too beautiful, that the beauty itself was ominous. The weather that day was definitely sunny and clear, the kind of early fall day that New York City gets only a couple of weeks of a year and showcases the city at its most photogenic, but to me that was more of a small grace on an otherwise horrible day than an omen. It was fine weather to do a lot of walking in, I suppose, but not so spectacular that it lent any meaning to the day. (It did, however, offer everybody in the city a very clear view of planes hitting the World Trade Center, which is why there is so much footage from so many rooftops of the attack.)

We spent a lot of time immersed in the beautiful weather as we walked uptown, but watching that man loosen his tie on 59th Street and dig into a salad in the sun was the first time that it even occurred to me that it was really nice out. There was something jarring about coming out of such a dramatic circumstance only to watch life go on as it normally would just a few miles uptown. Those people all knew what had happened by then and, probably correctly, judged that it did not involve them. They were as trapped by the shutdown trains as any of us, but their offices weren't covered in dust. They were probably thinking, *Thank God these other people got to safety.*

That's not to say that when they called their relatives later that night they didn't tell a different story, a dramatic tale about being mere blocks away from the towers and hurriedly evacuating. Many stories shifted in their retelling. Half of my family outside the city called the other half of my family to tell them I had been in danger, that they were personally affected. My cousins got a lot of credit in their middle and elementary school classrooms in New England for being related to me. I'm a little proud of that. But given how much lunch-time sunbathing was going on, 59th Street might as well have been Miami. At the same time, Miami didn't seem far enough away to feel truly safe.

The 59th Street Bridge was closed to traffic on one side so the thousands of pedestrians heading to Queens could take it by foot. I continued to follow Laura, vaguely aware that I was making an irreversible decision. Once on the bridge, I would not be able to turn back—there was no clear pathway among the thousands of evacuees for gawkers and indecisive kids who changed their minds and needed to head back into Manhattan. I felt a rush of adrenaline. I was not going home, that was now certain, and I was openly defying my parents. This wasn't something I did often or lightly. They were pretty easygoing and because of that I rarely broke rules. I wished, however, that they would read into my worry that they, too, should leave Manhattan. They seemed almost too calm about staying downtown.

On the bridge, another call came through on my phone, from my friend Indrina. She was, by then, at a Midtown office with family and another friend of ours. They were heading back to Queens, where she lived, and when she heard I was heading that way she told me that I could go to her house if I needed to.

Because we live at the center of so many things, people don't think of Manhattanites as being provincial, but we are in our own way. Growing up in Manhattan, especially in the days before Brooklyn was cool and everybody was priced out of anywhere convenient, I rarely went to the outer boroughs. Aside from family, people almost always came to you if you lived in "the city," the term outer-borough people use to reference Manhattan and Manhattan people use to reference the entire city.

At Stuyvesant I made a lot of friends from other parts of the city, but my borough ignorance continued. I have many good friends whom I've known for years, whose parents I've known for years, and yet whose houses I've been to less than a handful of times or not at all. Stuyvesant was, in fact, the first time I got the opportunity to develop close friendships with people from other boroughs, save a few childhood friends from places close to Manhattan like Brooklyn Heights. My father and three of my grandparents were born in Brooklyn, most of them were raised there for at least for some of their childhood, and yet, by age fourteen, I had no idea how to get to any neighborhood that wasn't directly across the river. Friendships at Stuyvesant had taught me a lot about navigating these unfamiliar parts of the city, but by senior year, Indrina's house was still the only place in Queens I would have known how to get to, and, frankly, I probably just barely would have made it. In going to Astoria, a neighborhood only a couple of stops into Queens, I was truly going into the unknown. Still, I told Indrina that I was okay. I was pretty sure Laura's parents would take me in. I warned her that if I lost Laura I might just show up at her door. She told me they'd be ready.

Laura and I stepped off the bridge into a mass of people all unsure of what their next transportation move was. We were tired—we'd walked for miles—and nobody had any reliable information about how the rest of the transit system was faring. With cell phone calls still difficult to make, we waited in a long line for a pay phone and each called our parents. Laura told hers that she was bringing a friend home and, thankfully, they were happy to accommodate. I called my dad, who, this time more forcefully, told me to turn around, walk back across the bridge, and come home. He didn't know how laughable his command seemed to me as I watched a stampede moving in from the opposite direction; he was just trying to wrestle some control back from an outlandish situation. Once again I stood my ground, uncharacteristically defiant. I told him I wouldn't be returning to Manhattan and that I'd call again from Laura's house. I'm sure it wasn't comforting that he had no idea who Laura was—I wasn't even entirely sure where she lived, so I just kept repeating that I was going to Astoria and finally hung up the phone. My mom, who was working at her school in Midtown and busy trying to reunite little kids with their parents, didn't hear about any of these conversations until later.

Neither Laura nor I am positive how we got back to her house from the bridge. I remember us riding a city bus, but she swears she wouldn't have known how to do that and instead remembers her brother driving down to pick us up. Either way, that ride was when it occurred to me that my feet really hurt. That's because, among the obstacles I had created for myself in insisting on walking far out of my way—all the way to Queens—there was the fact that I'd worn new shoes.

The shoes, the silver ones with Velcro straps, had, at seventeen, seemed rebellious and ironic. *Velcro! For an almost adult!* I've never been a fantastic dresser, and certainly high school was not a highlight among the many eras of my mediocre fashion sense, but I loved those shoes, their flashy metallic sheen. And after that initial walk, which began with a national tragedy and ended with tragic blisters, they were perfectly broken in and incredibly comfortable.

I wore the shoes for the rest of that year, not really thinking about their symbolic significance, but after I replaced them my mother put them in storage, relics of the era. She still has them somewhere, likely the only items in my parents' house that are still contaminated with WTC dust nearly twenty years later. Mice or roaches or some other brand of ubiquitous New York City critter has probably gotten cancer from them by now. Once, years later, I found them in the back of a closet, stiff and brittle. I guess WTC dust isn't great for leather either.

ONCE WE WERE SAFELY ensconced on a cute residential block on the far side of Astoria, Laura's house turned out to be the perfect place to hide out at the end of a long day of evacuating. Laura's parents fed us, comforted us, and handed me the phone so I could call my parents, who had been anxiously awaiting further news. I let them know I was safe and fed, and we made a plan to get me home the next day. Laura's older brother was going to take the train with me into the city on his way to a college course. It was the kind of plan you make for a ten-year-old, though I was seventeen. He was only twenty-three, not exactly a dyed-in-the-wool adult.

Laura also had a younger brother who was a Stuy student, a freshman, and wasn't home yet when we got there. Laura says she still feels guilty that she didn't think to find him at school before the evacuations began. I don't remember how he got home, but he showed up a little while after us, exhausted but fine. City kids are pretty resourceful.

That evening we all watched the news together and, like much of America, saw the word "terrorism" change before our eyes. On the morning of September 11, "terrorist" was a generic descriptor I would have applied to anybody who intentionally did something violent. I might have called the WTC attack a terrorist attack, but without meaning to imply any particular brand of violence or extremism. Even during my evacuation and walk uptown, if you'd asked me what a terrorist was, I'd have named a famous domestic terrorist like Ted Kaczynski, the Unabomber. When I walked into Laura's house my only point of comparison for who might do something as dramatic as plot for months and literally learn how to fly airplanes to take down the World Trade Center was Timothy McVeigh, the man responsible for the Oklahoma City bombing, an act of domestic terror that killed 168 people and injured over 650 others in 1995.[12] In my teenage experience, terrorism was American-made. It was the purview of white middle-aged men.

By the time we turned on the news that night, the entire nation seemed to agree that "terrorism" meant something much more specific now, a certain brand of Islamic extremism. It was a shift in perception that negatively impacted many people, including many of my classmates. Laura and I were able to walk for miles without incident. People were kind to us during the walk uptown, as we made our way over the bridge, and in the pay phone line. A lot of Stuyvesant students evacuated in less fortuitous circumstances. By the time we'd gotten to Laura's house, multiple classmates of ours traveling through other parts of the city had fielded slurs simply for looking vaguely Middle Eastern or South Asian. Some were called terrorists, while others were told to "go back to their country." It was an atrocious burden to put on a bunch of New York City teenagers who were, like us, just trying to figure out how to get home when the trains weren't running. Their evacuation gave them a crash course in how the dialogue had changed since 8:46 that morning, something I was able to remain blissfully unaware of until I was sitting in front of a television that night. Still, we all got the message eventually, and the change in our understanding of what "terrorism" was and who "terrorists" were took hold rapidly. By the next day, the definitions seemed settled. Our political dialogue had already entered a new and terrifying phase.

On the news that night, videos of the disaster played over and over, punctuated by a few speculative photos of Osama bin Laden and accompanied by a running ticker of the names of missing people—a never-ending stream of morbid question marks. The early footage of the first plane hitting was all amateur stuff taken from random rooftops, but eventually professional crews with helicopters took over the recording. The collapse of the towers, aside from being the most videotaped disaster ever at that point, had so much coverage from every vantage point that it could be edited together to look like it was the brainchild of a Hollywood studio, not a bunch of religious extremists. The sheer amount of video footage the news was able to play was still pretty novel at that point—it was before smartphones turned everybody into an amateur news reporter. For a long time, I couldn't tear myself away from the TV and the endless loops of video, which seems crazy now considering I haven't been able to stomach watching the collapse of the towers in the years since. I watched enough to last a lifetime that day. The more I saw, the more bizarre it felt. The more distant it became. That was, oddly, comforting.

FOR A LONG TIME, my memories of 1998's infamous freshman fires were essentially wiped out by September 11. I didn't think about them again until years later. The story of 9/11 was so distracting that nobody had any reason to ask about my high school experience before 2001. It was like the world had pushed a reset button that wiped out my childhood and ushered me into the cold, hard adult world where evacuations weren't just fun and games anymore.

The election, the thing I'd been most concerned about that morning, wound up being postponed to later in the month. On the day of the rescheduled mayoral primary, I'm sure I watched returns and gossiped and griped and complained, but I don't particularly remember it, nor do I remember much about how Michael Bloomberg got elected mayor that November beyond the fact that it was close and that, by that point, the electoral environment felt more tribal than substantive. Outside of Lower Manhattan the political narrative had shifted in an instant, and a lot of the silliness of that primary season had already dissolved into stoic speeches about security and the politics of fear. None of that was particularly helpful to us.

I didn't get to vote in the rescheduled election, but starting on that September day in 2001, city policy began to play a major role in my life. It greatly impacted the ways in which the WTC disaster carried forward for me and my classmates, and it certainly had an impact on our worldview. I'm still frustrated that I didn't have a say in these changes.

Though so much about that mayoral race got lost in the fog of the disaster, when I wake up on the anniversary of September 11 now, my first thought is always about that election—rather, how that election would end up having a direct impact on my life. At the time I still thought of voting as a fun civic celebration and not much else. But yes, I admit, I also think about how the weather that day was beautiful. Those people are right too.

CHAPTER 2

FLEEING

On the morning of September 12, Laura's older brother rode the train back to Manhattan with me. His college classes on the Upper East Side had, optimistically, not been canceled despite the mass exodus from Manhattan the day before. Hunter College's administrators were apparently the kind of confident, above-59th-Street people who knew the acrid smell in the air downtown and hazy view down Lexington Avenue wasn't their problem to solve. My parents met me outside the 68th Street subway station wearing supportive smiles pasted onto blank stares, a look that was common among New Yorkers in that first twenty-four hours after the attacks. I was nervous to see them given how much my life had changed in the last day and how sure I was that they didn't fully understand that change. They seemed nervous to see me too.

We walked home from 68th Street, two miles of evolving panic at every noise, jostle, and subway passage underneath. The smell of the air, thick with a smoky, artificial, hard-to-place stench, got worse with each passing block. It's disquieting to walk toward a dangerous smell and know you'll never pass to fresh air on the other side. With my parents there I couldn't follow my strong instinct to turn around and head back toward the clear sky, so I kept drifting ahead toward an amorphous white haze. All three of us stared into the gulf reluctantly, unsure of where its margins began and ended and whether we'd already been enveloped by them.

One of the odd things about living in such an expansive and densely populated city is that each neighborhood reacts to sudden change in its own way. I had noticed this the day before as Laura and I passed those lunch breakers luxuriating in the sun at outdoor cafés in Midtown as we rushed by, still stunned and afraid. I noticed it again on the twelfth. The city seemed to break down like this: People above 42nd Street, removed just enough from the madness downtown, went about their business, buying their coffees and newspapers, rushing down the street in suits, carrying heavy work bags, and wearing uncomfortable shoes. People below 42nd Street and the now empty expanse of Times Square were more uneasy. They stared at the top of the Empire State Building, visible high above the other buildings lining 34th Street, like it was some sort of malicious transformer that might blow at any moment. Others wandered through coffee shops posting signs picturing missing people. People below 34th Street didn't really know where they were or what they were supposed to be doing. I was happy to stop at 25th Street, though some people felt called to return even farther downtown to see what it looked like.

The only way to get behind the hastily constructed barricade at 14th Street was to live there or volunteer, and very little was being done to vet the volunteers. Some classmates of mine went down, were handed paper suits and crates of water, and then were given free rein to wander around the disaster area handing out supplies. At one point on the twelfth I did walk down to the 14th Street border with my parents, but I had no desire to go any farther, no real curiosity about how things looked in the dust zone. It was hard enough just to walk down the canyon of Sixth Avenue, which had perfectly framed the Twin Towers the day before and now framed a tall, never-ending tower of smoke.

Wherever they were, people were going about their business quietly, unceremoniously. Even as we trudged through Midtown the city felt oddly empty, though in truth many of us were stranded there. The bridges and tunnels were either gridlocked or closed and air traffic was grounded, so nearly everybody who had the misfortune of being in New York on the eleventh remained there on the twelfth.

When we arrived at my parents' house, I was somewhat shocked to find that our apartment was still the same. Books stacked three layers deep on our large living room shelves. Clothing still coating my bedroom chair. A thousand kinds of cheese mingling in the fridge. Something about the excessive normalcy felt unwarranted given the circumstances. There was only one aberration: messages from all over the country filled our answering machine. As I listened to them, it occurred to me that there were people out there who spent September 11 worried that I was dead. The situation was so serious that instead of wondering if I had spent the night in Queens, people were worried that I was trapped under a falling building.

The messages of concern did not compute to me. As the towers collapsed, I was thinking about taking action, about getting away, not about dying. Dying never occurred to me. In retrospect it was almost preferable to have had some agency in the situation—to not watch helplessly from Massachusetts, wondering whether people you cared about were gone, frustrated by your inability to save them.

Further phone messages inquired as to the fate of my school, where evidently a television reporter, amid the chaos, had set up shop and reported that a bomb threat was under investigation within the building.[13] I got several calls from family and friends in New Mexico, of all places, asking about this. The Southwest had apparently been on the case, watching out for suspicious activity at Stuyvesant High School despite the presence of myriad actual dangers that day.

Fortunately, I was long gone by the time a reporter decided to connect the extraordinary story of the Twin Towers crumbling with a vague threat of attack on New York City public schools, but I was happy to see that, despite my heightened state of fear, the bomb business still sounded absurd to me. It was reassuring to know that I had not lost all perspective.

My mother returned most of the calls to let people know that I was okay, but I do remember talking to my aunt and uncle, one of the numerous concerned calls from New Mexico. They wanted details—What could I see? What could I smell? Did I see the planes? Did I see people jump? Did I see people die? I think at the time they thought they were helping talk me through a trauma, but the call was so memorably upsetting and their questions so visceral and graphic that I suddenly felt an immediate and overwhelming need to drop the phone.

The realization that I simply could not narrate my experience hit me with such force that it surprised even me. I went silent for a few minutes, brain scrambling between replies that varied from shouting to throwing something to hanging up, and settled for repeating, "I don't want to talk about it," over and over and furiously waving the phone at my parents. I was having a hard enough time getting a handle on my anxiety without people asking me to have feelings about everything too. The awful smell that infil-trated the apartment served as a reminder that we were still in the process of dealing with something, protected in some part by shock. That call was what kept me away from the counselors at school in the weeks following. It kept me away from therapists for many years after. It took me fifteen years to seek out therapy for PTSD. I wasn't ready to talk about it until I was ready, and on September 12, I was, as it turned out, not ready.

Other calls offered condolences for my presumed losses. Oddly enough, I didn't know anybody firsthand who died in the attacks. I heard stories of secondhand cousins and mothers and friends and the like, but even though I was there, lived in Lower Manhattan, and ran from the event itself, working in the World Trade Center was not that common where I am from. I had never even gone up to the top, let alone visited an office there. Whole towns in New Jersey were decimated by the attacks, but I can't think of a single person from my community who was lost on that day. For us the deaths came later, all from illness. That scent in our homes had consequences. Bad air was our loss.

As is true after many extraordinary events, rumors of the urban-legend variety ran rampant for the next few weeks, testing our sense of reality in the face of this new systemic chaos. It was acceptable to spread these rumors to any person you knew, no matter how casually. According to several unreliable sources, somebody had surfed down the crumbling facade of the second tower on a desk and lived. According to others, somebody who jumped from the upper floors had landed in just the right way as to not be harmed. Then there were the stories of people on the ground dying after being hit by jumpers. Those were probably the only rumors that were true, but we tried to put stock in as many of the miraculous ones as we could. The rescue operation at the site was finding very few survivors, and we all needed a little hope.[14]

Neighborly conversations about 9/11 were, in part, a reaction to the constant visual reminders of disaster. The blocks surrounding my house, close to the police barricades blocking traffic into Lower Manhattan, transformed overnight and kept changing. Not only was the skyline different, but human-scale tokens of tragedy abounded. People searching for loved ones formed a line that wrapped around the block of an old armory down the street. Missing signs popped up everywhere, multiplying by the day. The faces of a startlingly diverse collection of people covered every fence, wall, and store window—anywhere there was space. The subjects in the pictures were smiling, not aware of their fate. One has to assume that many of the people in those early missing signs were found. We didn't know the extent of the human toll at the time, but the rolls of dead came from isolated parts of the WTC complex and the emergency response teams that went to save them. And what would that many children have been doing on the ninetieth floor of the towers during school hours anyway? What would an elderly man have been doing up there? Perhaps they were missing because our cell phones were not working. Perhaps they went home with friends instead of family. Perhaps.

Beyond the phone calls, there were other indications that I was right to avoid home the day before. Being there was wholly exhausting, much more so than being tucked away in Astoria. Not only were there many reminders of the events all around the neighborhood, but I was jumping ten feet at every sound in an area that was already a cacophony before fighter jets and other military aircraft began to pass overheard constantly. My anxiety, instead of subsiding from the comfort of being in familiar surroundings, was becoming more problematic. Every loud noise—and living on a mixed-use block, there was always noise—felt like a reminder that attacks could come out of nowhere. That Americans were no longer supposed to feel safe. That we were supposed to be "terrorized."

My parents continued to exhibit a lack of urgency that was frustrating, probably because they had adult things to worry about like jobs and whether my school would reopen. With nowhere to be, I went to my mother's school for a day and stoically watched the kindergarteners build tall towers out of blocks, then knock them down, mimicking what they'd seen on TV. Finally, two days into the post-9/11 period and after heavy lobbying from me, we packed up our car (how lucky to have a car!) and braved the bridges out of Manhattan. Our first trip across the George Washington Bridge in the post-terror world was grueling, not because of traffic but because of an intractable idea that implanted itself in my head the moment we were above water: *We could die here.* Not because I could see anything suspicious or hear anything loud. Just because, as I now knew, these things can happen out of the blue. It took hours for the smell of Ground Zero smoke to fully dissipate from our car and our clothing. My mother noted with shock that she was finally smelling fresh air as we passed through Monticello, New York, almost 100 miles from the city.

Our destination was a house my parents had purchased in upstate New York before they'd garnered the savings to buy an apartment in the city. It was in a town just outside the fashionable summer-home ring, three and a half hours by car into central New York State. My grandparents lived in the area as well, in an adorable craftsman house on the main drag of a village with no stoplight. As a rule, I generally tried to avoid trips to "the country" given my aversion to nature and gnawing quiet. I was, to be fair, also allergic to the entire region. That house was the site of many childhood asthma attacks that turned into ER visits. It was a place I had never enjoyed clearheaded because there was pollen in the summer and dusty, closed-up house musk in the winter, and when all of those make your eyes itch, New York City seems like a wondrous bastion of clean air and health. No more. Central New York was finally where the clean air was. When we got up there, I told myself, *We are finally somewhere so random that no person would think to attack us.* A better Astoria.

The fact that upstate residents, to my mind, did not have to worry about being attacked made their panicked frenzy endearing. To them 9/11 was a symbolic act of violence to be incensed about, not an experience to recall fearfully. The widespread concern for me in town made me feel like my ability to feel safe at school was important to them. Like I was important to them. Like they did not hate city folks as much as people said.

As soon as we got to our corner of "the country," we immediately went to visit with my grandparents. My grandfather, a veteran of World War II who had raised four girls in the Vietnam era, took a look at me in my shell-shocked state and said, "We're the only two members of the family who have been to war." I don't pretend that's true—while we were both "drafted" in a sense, he was away fighting for years, even missing my mom's birth. He got shot at and freed concentration camps. I abandoned a bunch of kids in wheelchairs and ran away from something I wasn't personally involved in.

I did, however, understand his war experiences differently from that point on. Prior to that visit, I had never been that interested in war stories. In history class war seemed like a purely theoretical phenomenon, one in which men visit needless violence upon other men in an effort to look heroic, usually under the presumed banner of a noble cause. My grandfather had, at times, tried to relay a more human-scale story of war. At one point he wrote a series of letters to me and my cousins detailing his World War II experiences in a serialized fashion. I'd read the letters with mild disinterest, almost like they were homework. After 9/11, however, in the same way that sometimes a book or a movie can help you experience a historical event on an instinctive level instead of on an intellectual one, I started to think about my grandfather's World War II experiences with an autogenous understanding of what it's like to face a danger that's too big to see the full shape of. Also, of what it's like to pass days, months, even years in a state of heightened fear.

Once upstate, my parents and I spent a few days trying to create some sort of routine, but after a while the stillness became a problem. I felt a nervous need to be on the move. We began looking for activities to fill our time, eventually landing on something very typically appealing to a Stuyvesant family—we went to visit colleges, specifically colleges that were outside of the tristate area and therefore in little danger of being attacked by terrorists. (Most of my travel plans for the next year were based on this criterion.) The college trips were intended to reaffirm my sense of normalcy. I had spent three years thinking of nothing but the ways in which college could make or break my life. I wanted to get back to being nervous about the right stuff.

At the time, I had a few must-haves for my college, most of them ridiculous. I wanted my school to have hardwood floors in the dorms (I care about my living space, so sue me), a politically progressive reputation (so I'd have friends to protest with), good ice cream in the cafeteria (only the Vermont schools came out strong in that category), and, embarrassingly enough coming from a math-and-science high school student, limited requirements in math and science. On September 12, I had added a new criterion that trumped the rest: an exceptionally random location. As a result of my new top priority, some unexpected colleges began to look very enticing. As we drove up to the remote campuses that made up our tour, I began to see trees differently, less as allergy and boredom factories and more as protection. My visual comprehension of the world was changing.

Even in the middle of nowhere, however, it turned out that it wasn't easy to outrun the World Trade Center. At every turn, in every lull, in every moment, 9/11 interjected itself. Haverford College's art gallery was named for Cantor Fitzgerald, a company located at the top of the World Trade Center's North Tower that lost nearly their entire staff, 658 people, in that one foul act.[15] That the Pennsylvania liberal arts college didn't have a sign up in the gallery noting this was an offense I could not get over for the entire length of the tour. Other schools didn't seem to get the enormity of the events, ignoring them so we would remember their campus as cheerful and focus on how many a cappella groups they offered. At Williams College in western Massachusetts I cried, surprising myself, when I realized that I might not be able to access my transcript by the application deadline. Stuyvesant was being used as a command center, and we were getting news that we'd be displaced for some time. The admissions lady comforted me, implying that, frankly, even without grades, Stuyvesant students were going to get into whatever colleges they wanted.

It was on the Haverford College tour that the first mention of war came up. Haverford, an old Quaker outpost with an educational tradition rooted in pacifism, evidently employs future military types as tour guides. In addressing the events of 9/11, our guide led us to a shady tree, sat on a brick fence, and in the contrived dramatic tone that is necessary in these moments, told us that his friends had all agreed that they would enlist should America decide to go to war over the World Trade Center. They didn't want to abandon the nation in its time of need.

I still wonder what drove those well-educated young men to fantasize about enlisting. Surely, they were not so blindly drawn into the political fervor surrounding America's various invasions that they would give up their idyllic, civilized lives in a pacifist corner of Pennsylvania—all in the name of patriotism? Who would be left to sing in those a cappella concerts? Or drunkenly misquote Sartre at dorm parties? Or strum along to Elliot

Smith songs on the quad?

I, for one, was not ready to face the concept of future violence after my own world had been so shattered by it, and I was certainly not ready to hear the drumbeat to war while visiting a Quaker college. I decided against Haverford in that moment.

MY OBSESSION WITH BEING outside of the city as the recovery efforts continued meant that I was out of town during the Great Mural Project of 2001. On September 16, a Stuyvesant student's mother purchased a few tarps and buckets of paint and invited the Stuyvesant community to meet in a park downtown and paint murals.[16] My friends talked about the project ad nauseam, probably because it was the first time any of them got to be real teenagers that week. We'd all been trapped at home with our parents for days. Everything even an inch outside our homes was feared as too dangerous, especially for many of my Arab and South Asian friends, who were starting to get profiled, slurred at, or threatened wherever they went. Additionally, very few of our parents understood the true extent of what we'd witnessed, knew how to talk to us about 9/11, or, most importantly, knew *not* to talk to us about 9/11. Spending some time with people who understood not just the trauma of evacuation but what it had been like to live with that trauma since was probably as healing as the chance to exorcise some anxiety via paintbrush.

The murals were hanging outside on the day we returned to Stuyvesant a few weeks later, there to remind us of the unity that the students who painted them ostensibly felt in that park. To me they were more of a question mark because, no matter how hard I looked at them, I couldn't quite figure out what they were supposed to show. They were not the only murals adorning the school that day. There is a great artistic tradition of schools sending aesthetically questionable projects to other schools as a show of solidarity. Stuyvesant was blanketed in murals for weeks.

During the mural week I also missed an expedition to Lower Manhattan that three of my closest friends took to visit the office of one of their fathers. I'm not sure how or why this excursion came together—in its retelling it sounded a bit like typical teenager herd thinking, as if once two people had signed on, everybody had to go. Nobody had anything else to do anyway. The trio later told me that they were glad I hadn't joined. The air was so thick with smoke and dust down by the Financial District that, with my asthma, I would have had to turn back anyway. They held handkerchiefs over their mouths and noses, makeshift protection that was probably more a mental salve than a physical one.

The one excursion I didn't miss out on was a group appearance on *The Montel Williams Show*, a cheesy daytime talk show that I'd never watched a full episode of, with those same three friends. We taped it on September 17, the day I returned from my college tour upstate. We all met at my house, and the show sent a limousine to pick us up—an unusual thrill that was simultaneously exciting and disorienting. I felt displaced, but also very fancy and important. There was no audience at the taping, just a panel of other kids from New York and New Jersey that we sat at the center of. I don't remember what was said when the cameras were on—I think our foursome sucked up a lot of the air in the room, interrupting other people's comments, boisterously waving our hands at the producers like the eager students we were—but I distinctly remember the way we vehemently argued with Montel during the commercial breaks. We pestered him about whether he thought we should retaliate militarily for the attacks of the prior week. We told him he didn't know what he was talking about when he said he did. We told him we were the ones who knew what it was to live with the consequences. When the episode aired, we bristled about how cheesy and reductive the final edit had been. How it didn't really tell our story. We knew Montel wasn't famous for doing deep dives into complicated political issues, but something about his trite depiction of us and our experience stung anyway. Later, though my friends talked frequently about the mural project and their dangerous walk downtown, we seemed to silently agree we'd let our memories block out the Montel experience. Even now, when periodically one of us will ask the group, "Remember when we did *Montel*?" the collective answer is almost always, "I completely forgot about that."

Even though I'd made it back to New York in time for the *Montel* taping, I was a little bit jealous of some of my friends' experiences in that first week after the attacks, of the formative memories they had made. I suffer from a fear of missing out, or FOMO, as much as anybody. In retrospect, however, I respect that my priority in that first week after 9/11 was to be outside of the city. For some reason I had the strongest need to get off the island of anybody I knew, and despite my teenage insecurity and my resulting willingness to doubt my own feelings in most circumstances, I remain proud of the fact that I took my needs seriously and did what I needed to do, FOMO be damned. At the time I worried I was overreacting, but I don't regret that either. My overreaction was validated later because, while we were upstate, the head of the Environmental Protection Agency, Christine Todd Whitman, made a choice that would have consequences for the federal government for decades to come. On September 14, the *New York Daily News* published an article with the headline "EPA Chief Says Water and Air Are Safe."[17] Those initial comments were made while I was poking around at colleges, safely ensconced in the trees of upstate New York. On September 18,[18] the day after I returned to the city, Whitman released a written statement that said: "I am glad to reassure the people of New York and Washington, DC, that their air is safe to breathe and their water is safe to drink."[19] Those declarations from the EPA chief set in motion a series of events that would later make hundreds of thousands of people sick.

CHAPTER 3

BROOKLYN

I returned to the city right before school started back up. Stuyvesant's official student website, www.stuynet.com, was down, so our reporting instructions came through a phone tree from the administration and a student-run spoof website called www.stuycom.net, which had been built the year before by Gary He, a student infamous for his gift with computers and causing trouble. The site was not only unaffiliated with the administration but had, on various occasions, been at odds with the principal and several of his underlings. After 9/11, with no social media yet in the mix and no access to most official channels of information, www.stuycom.net was our main source of information and how most of the student body found out we were to report to another one of the large science schools, Brooklyn Tech.

Brooklyn Tech is, as it happens, in Brooklyn. True to my provincial Manhattanite upbringing, I had no idea how to get there. On the day of our first big back to school meeting in the Brooklyn Tech auditorium, I met a friend in the subway so that neither of us would get lost alone, and we watched the butchered Manhattan skyline with amazement as our subway flew over the Williamsburg Bridge, a cloud of smoke hovering over the Financial District. Every time I saw this I felt a great sense of relief. Getting off the island continued to hold appeal.

Brooklyn Tech turned out to be an imposing deco-era building in Fort Greene, Brooklyn, that hovered ponderously over a small neighborhood of historic row houses, independent shops, and small cafés. My only point of reference when I first arrived was that it was down the block from Junior's, a diner offering the city's most famous cheesecake.

At that initial meeting, we heard a few contradictory things about what our school schedule would be like moving forward. The principal initially said the plan was to run something like twenty classes at once in the school theater, then find space for the rest of us where they could. As soon as students began to file in, however, it was clear that holding even two classes in that old Board of Education theater, filled with wooden furniture and prone to echo, would be a stretch. As one speaker attempted to compete with the voices of thousands of teenagers chattering among themselves, the wheels began to spin in various administrator heads. They quickly realized they would need to find a different compromise to teach the five thousand Brooklyn Tech and three thousand Stuyvesant students now competing for space in the building. Because of the confusion, I didn't glean much from the experience about what our day-to-day would become or how I should feel about it. The meeting ended rather abruptly with a speech from our student body president, and then something odd: the Pledge of Allegiance.

Every school system deals with the Pledge differently, but at that time in New York City, students generally stopped reciting it by the end of elementary school. The last time I had heard the Pledge of Allegiance was in first grade, when I had gotten in trouble for not saying "under God." My mother had informed me that I didn't have to say the words, but evidently my omission was seen as a source of great controversy at my school. My teacher asked my mother about it specifically at parent-teacher night, and my mother confirmed that she had allowed me that privilege. We did not, in fact, believe in God. My teacher, a very religious woman herself, had taken it in stride.

By 2001, I had gone one better. I was an experienced protester of many things by that time—impeachments, military actions, cuts to union benefits—and I had learned that another thing those of us "in the know" could do to express dismay with our nation's direction was to sit down during the Pledge. On that September day in 2001, President Bush was already talking about going to war, conspiracy theories about 9/11 abounded, and I was angry with the way this terrifying event had been used by public officials to create an environment of fear that would justify stripping people of their rights, so I remained seated. When I was pressed about it by a nearby teacher, my explanation sounded stronger than I expected. Without giving her the context, I just said, "I don't stand for the Pledge," like it was a blanket rule. It was an off-the-cuff statement that began a revolution.

Or so I thought. For years, I believed I was the only person to sit in that large meeting. The only person during a time of great national unity and tragedy to forgo allegiance to a piece of cloth in a nation that had, as it turned out, deceived me. Years later I found out that a few friends, all disconnected from each other and in different enough social circles that our stories about this didn't cross for a long time, also claim to be the only person who sat for the Pledge in that meeting. I couldn't see anybody else sitting from where I sat, and I'm sure we all felt equally alone as we did it, but it's nice to know we actually did it as a team, even if after the fact. I was not even the bravest person to attempt it—one of the students who sat is a Muslim American classmate of mine who, after losing family in the towers and, frankly, his feeling of safety as he began receiving side-eye in the subway and racist comments on the street just for being brown, simply thought "not today."

Either way, whether or not I was the only person to sit in that September meeting, I was certainly not the only person to end the year seated for the Pledge. By the time we went to war, half of my class would remain seated for it every day. Friends who weren't much for protesting even found themselves seated in the hallway or other inconvenient locations if that became necessary. By the end of the year, standing for the Pledge was what made a statement.

THE SCHEDULE WE FINALLY did settle on for sharing the Brooklyn Tech building was an uneasy compromise at best—Brooklyn Tech students would do a morning shift, and Stuyvesant kids would attend in the afternoon. Classes would be about twenty minutes long, and school would start at 7:00 a.m. for them and end around 5:00 p.m. for us.

It didn't help that, for most of their history, Brooklyn Tech and Stuyvesant have had a somewhat adversarial relationship. They continue to use the same admissions exam: Stuyvesant takes the eight hundred highest-scoring students, and Brooklyn Tech admits the third tier of scorers. Truth be told, the competition is primarily one-sided. Stuyvesant students generally assume they attend the best school in the city and rarely interrogate this notion of the "best" further. Other schools, in turn, all claim that they are Stuyvesant's one and only true rival. We're arrogant—what can I say? As soon as I started college, I was told by alumni of no fewer than four city schools that they had attended Stuyvesant's biggest rival. I learned to smile and nod. All of these schools, Stuyvesant included, perform roughly as well as each other anyway. There isn't really a "best."

With that said, the degree to which the Stuyvesant student body's aloofness was irritating to students at other schools was never clear to me, in fact had never ever occurred to me, until we were sharing a building with "our biggest rival" in Brooklyn. Brooklyn Tech students seemed bigger, there were more of them, and they were cranky because thanks to our presence their school day began at 7:00 a.m. (not the ideal schedule for five thousand teenagers). The tension was palpable on the way to school as we walked toward the building in a three-thousand-person phalanx and past the Brooklyn Tech student body leaving for the day. Stories of bullying began to spread. Many of us avoided eye contact with anybody walking in the opposite direction as we trudged our way from the DeKalb Avenue subway station toward our temporary home. It was like living Jane Elliott's infamous experiment[20] in which she'd split third-graders up by eye color and then assign one group an arbitrary privilege or distinction. We were nearly identical groups of nerdy math and science kids, trudging to and from the same kind of nerdy math and science school, and we were vaguely aware that we should hate each other, but the distinction was arbitrary. Like Stuyvesant, Brooklyn Tech is also a school for academically gifted city kids who scored well on a standardized exam. We were meaningfully the same, aside from the sour note of trauma and anxiety that we Stuyvesant kids were bringing to the table.

Brooklyn Tech students did have more minor reasons to be irritated with us. Complaints about the lack of amenities in their building made it to their ears alarmingly quickly. Brooklyn Tech is housed in a traditional NYC Board of Education monolith with ten stories accessed by too many stairs, a meandering downtrodden-looking cafeteria, and several classrooms that looked like sawmills and factory boiler rooms. Stuyvesant students—who were accustomed to a lux early nineties edifice with escalators to help battle those ten-story hikes, a beautiful cafeteria that overlooked the Hudson River, a new swimming pool, state-of-the-art science laboratories, robotics labs, new drafting equipment, and zero classrooms that look like mills— were not always gracious guests.

To me, however, and possibly only to me, Brooklyn Tech was thrilling. I was one of the few students who loved wandering the building. I've long been entranced by the impressively grand and once groundbreaking architectural features of New York City's older school buildings. Mr. Scotti's architecture class, despite its unceremonious ending on the eleventh, was made more interesting by our brief recess at Tech. The drafting and architecture classroom felt like a history lesson on the culture and design aesthetic of the 1930s, when immovable wooden drafting boards and male students in suits and ties were what composed technical education. Ditto for the science labs, which were fun to explore because of their museum-like quality. (None of us ever considered the challenges of having to do an experiment in them. Our classes were so short we didn't have time anyway.)

I also fulfilled a personal mission in those weeks, finally attending a school with the original bronze NYC Board of Education doorknobs still in commission. I had developed an obsession with these after my uncle gifted my parents a replica of one. It was in use on the bathroom door of our apartment for most of my childhood. It wasn't rare to find a school in the city that still had them in use, but it felt rare to me because I had never gotten to attend one. My middle and elementary school were housed in the same 1960s building, designed long after flourishes like special public agency brassware were phased out. By the sixties, the city was apparently enamored with a jail aesthetic instead of bespoke custom hardware.

I was also fascinated by what I called the "mill" rooms and would sometimes wander the halls during my twenty-minute lunch period to look for them. Our college advisor's makeshift office, where seniors at Stuyvesant spent significant amounts of time attending meetings and seeking advice, was located in one of these rooms, with unused heavy machinery sitting silently behind two folding desks. Because of this unorthodox setup, there was no way to hold meetings with college reps. An admissions officer from Vassar, which would later become my college, came to visit at one point, and we found ourselves wandering the halls aimlessly, looking for a room in which to meet and questioning what there was even left to discuss.

In the interview, he waited for me to start. All I could think of was, *Hi, I'm a mess and likely won't recover my normal self until after beginning college so just know: I'm a little bit of a wild card.*

He seemed overwhelmed too, not sure what kind of scene he'd just walked into. The hallways were filled with zombie-like students. The administrators had no helpful resources for him. They couldn't even offer him a room in which to conduct his business.

Wisely, I stayed largely quiet during our mobile meeting and focused on questions I knew were appropriate, like "How many clubs do you offer?" Questions that had no relevance to my life at that moment and whose answers were of no interest to me. He answered them all in a forced cheery tone, relieved to launch into one of his preplanned spiels, relieved not to have to address head-on the bizarre environment and distressed students in front of him.

The college application process was greatly complicated by the Brooklyn Tech period for other reasons as well. For one thing, we were supposed to be getting our college recommendations finalized during that time. The school randomly assigned specific teachers to write SSRs, or Secondary School Reports, general school recommendations written for each student by a group of unlucky teachers. My SSR writer had to be switched late in the game because the original teacher I was assigned to, a Spanish teacher whose class I'd never taken, refused to include any information about my work related to Cuba. This work was pretty central to my plan to look like I had extracurriculars and was a well-rounded and interesting person. I had been working in the summers at a nonprofit called the Center for Cuban Studies, which organized legal trips to Cuba and housed a gallery with an extensive collection of Cuban art. I'd also gone on a trip to Cuba the summer before and started a club at school called the Action for Cuba Club. The club had four members and no real track record of doing anything, but an extracurricular on paper was good enough for colleges, so it was good enough for me.

My original SSR writer had said that my work, because it implied that I opposed the US travel ban and embargo against Cuba, would ruin my chances of getting into the University of Miami, a school I wasn't considering applying to. I argued back. Then he suggested I could get an admissions officer of Cuban descent at any school and get rejected. I said I would take my chances, and my mom called the school to complain. I was soon switched to Annie Thoms, a young English teacher who was probably barely holding it together herself but met with me during those weeks in a random Brooklyn Tech office because we were so far behind. She gave me some brief comfort. Even if the world was falling apart, the SSR situation was finally under control.

Beyond the private doorknob and SSR-related benefits to me, there were a couple of larger upsides to the Brooklyn Tech era as well. Most important was that the Stuyvesant student body's school day did not start until 1:00 p.m. We were, for once, getting enough sleep. Additionally, our classes were shortened to the point of futility and our days were spent primarily complaining about frivolous things like the stairs and the fact that we could not leave the building for "lunch," which was actually an inconvenient twenty-minute period in the late afternoon, long past an actual mealtime.

The widespread unease emanating from every corner of the city gave us license to leave behind a few of our less time-sensitive obsessions with college and grades as well. The lack of academic pressure was a godsend at that unique moment, an era during which an entire class could be thrown to pieces by the noise of a motorcycle starting or car backfiring. At any sign of activity outside, students would jump up to look out the window and identify the source, hoping to assure themselves that it was not a malicious threat to our safety. Teachers, too, were at a bit of a loss. Some tried to carry on as if everything was normal, and others were clearly so shaken themselves that teaching was only barely on their minds.

The lack of pressure, in turn, gave us time to compensate for our stress by having fun. One day a good friend kidnapped me at the end of school and brought me to a Yankees game, something previously unheard of on a weeknight. People threw weeknight parties and parents acquiesced to demands from their children to allow them to stay out late on Tuesdays, which we began to refer to, not exactly cleverly, as "party night." By the time we had been at Brooklyn Tech for a couple of weeks, we really were lightening up, so it was with a mixed sense of dread and excitement that many of us learned that the Parents' Association was brokering a deal that would return us to Stuyvesant.

In those first few weeks post-9/11 there was, unsurprisingly, an immediate desire to get things back to normal that took hold all over the nation. Some of that was coming from outside—the rest of America, CEOs especially, wanted to get back to their regularly scheduled programming—but some of the agitation to return to normal also stemmed from local exhaustion. Everything had been too loud and scary and weird for too many days. People downtown were displaced from their homes, the financial sector was reeling because nobody could return to their Wall Street offices, and Chinatown's street economy was in shambles because nobody was shopping. It didn't help that the general mentality of New Yorkers even after a major event like 9/11 is to stand up in the face of the fear and anger and resolutely continue our lives.

In retrospect, I don't recommend this strategy. When the Environmental Protection Agency administrator Christie Todd Whitman made her infamous mid-September comments about the safety of the air downtown, it was long before the Environmental Protection Agency had any conclusive data on that point.[21] Nevertheless, other government agencies understood the comments as a federal mandate to resume normal life.[22] Whitman's boss's actions made additionally clear where the government's priorities lay. Amid news articles with headlines like "E.P.A. Says Air Is Safe, But Public Is Doubtful"[23] was news of President Bush meeting with business leaders and Chinatown schoolchildren to reassure consumers and families that things would get back to normal quickly.[24]

Thanks to the pressure from up high, local politicians started to echo Whitman's safety claims as well, eager to get the reeling downtown economy back on its feet. On September 18, the same day the EPA first put in writing that it was "safe to breathe,"[25] Mayor Giuliani made a show of returning to City Hall, just blocks from the towers, and declaring, "Now we are going to get back to work."[26] All but six of the city's schools reopened, and President

Bush called the NYC Schools chancellor, Harold Levy, and praised him for getting the schools up and running so quickly: "Your school system suffered, you picked yourself up, you got your students readjusted, resituated, and you're educating."[27]

The credibility the EPA's declaration lent to the reopening mission was critical. On September 17 the stock market was reopened, needlessly sending thousands of workers into the contamination zone.[28] Hundreds of thousands of unsuspecting people returned to their dusty downtown addresses starting in mid-September,[29] and when the city got pushback from people concerned that something didn't smell right down there, Stuyvesant students were brought in to put on a show. As the head of the Stuyvesant Parents' Association at the time, Marilena Christodoulou, put it to *The New York Times* just before our return, "Now Stuyvesant is seen as a symbol. There is tremendous political pressure to get us in there, because if it's safe for us to move in, then it is safe everywhere. Yes, we want to go back, but only when it is safe."[30]

By the time our tenure at Brooklyn Tech came to an end, the wisdom of returning to Stuyvesant's downtown building had become a source of major controversy among the student body. It was with a little shock and a lot of personal dread on my part that we received an official date for our return: October 9. Less than a month after the attacks. Plenty of students applauded the move, craving normalcy. Living downtown, however, I had my doubts about how safe it would be. It turned out I was right to.

CHAPTER 4

RETURN TO STUYVESANT

They opened up Chambers Street for us.

Before, that small stretch at the border of Tribeca and the western edge of the Financial District had been populated by National Guardsmen, who hesitantly allowed a couple of residents to sneak into their homes by inspecting pieces of their mail and comparing them to their IDs. Everybody else gathered on the far side of the barricades, craning their necks for glimpses of the tragedy beyond. Nearby, a few office workers—those whose companies didn't want to let a little smoke get in the way of moneymaking—filed into work.

On October 9 I stood at the top of the Chambers Street subway station stairs for a long time, nervously watching other high school students pass, some in dust masks, others shielding their mouths and noses with scarves, but most just breathing in the crisp morning air as if they couldn't smell the acrid stench. It reeked like a campfire mixed with a burning chemical plant. I've never smelled anything like it before or since, but whatever it was, it was much more concentrated than the periodic whiffs of smoke I'd inhaled from my home on 25th Street. It made you cough.

It was a long walk to the river, longer than usual thanks to the many checkpoints we passed, the reporters we fielded questions from, and the new sites we tiptoed over the rest of the herd to see. Bottlenecking began about one hundred feet before Greenwich Street, usually an unremarkable stoplight, a school on one side, residential buildings on the other, and a line of people at the McDonald's on the corner, waiting for their morning heart attack on a plate. The view on October 9, 2001, was different. For once, we were drawn to look south, where two metal girders smoked atop a pile of rubble, perfectly framed by the buildings on either side. It was a showstopping disaster-footage moment simultaneously highlighting what we were in for and what we had seen.

By the start of October, the excessive television coverage of the towers falling had interfered with much of my actual memory of the day. I did not just identify with running from the towers' collapse, as I had in real life, but I also pictured myself in the dust cloud and, somehow, filming from a nearby roof and casually commenting on how "big" this was. My overexposure to the footage had slowly allowed my own experience to drift into the realm of television, as if it were a distant action sequence, a memory that I needn't be trapped by. Greenwich Street was unquestionably real, however. It was a harsh signal that my memory of the day the towers fell wasn't the only thing tying me to it. One can compartmentalize the past, tuck it away so that it is possible to go on, but the present is urgent, unquestionably there. It can't be mixed up with television and dismissed.

The National Guardsmen posted at Greenwich Street, who despite being clad in heavy tactical gear still looked like a bunch of alarmed upstate boys scared enough at being in the city let alone at Ground Zero, hustled us along. No staring allowed. We were to march forward as if nothing of note was happening. A couple of days later they attempted to stop the pedestrian pileup at the intersection by stringing a large white sheet across the buildings on the south side, blocking the view of Ground Zero. The sheet had holes so that it wouldn't be blown off by the wind, however, and instead of blocking the view, the holes turned the panorama into a different kind of site, offering sudden, disturbing glimpses at unexpected intervals.

The plan to discourage gawkers didn't last long. People were going to look, after all. Those steel girders were celebrities by this point. Plus, there was a fire burning down there, and smoke was creeping up above the sheet, too high to block.

Slowly, hesitantly, we pushed on toward the school, showing our IDs at NYPD and National Guard checkpoints several times along the way until we finally stood at the familiar site of the footbridge that passes over West Street and leads into the Stuyvesant building. A truck full of debris passed underfoot as I made my way toward the front doors.

CITY OFFICIALS ASSURED US of many things as we prepared to return to Stuyvesant. The air was safe despite the fires that continued to burn at Ground Zero. The school was safe despite rampant reports that it had not been adequately cleaned. Most importantly, we were among guards and chaplains and therapists, should we suffer some sort of mental or physical harm. We were encouraged to seek help in the guidance office, now populated by specialized therapists holding group sessions. We could skip any class to go to one of these sessions. Any class we wanted. Even math.

Along with the assurances, however, was a new sign posted at the front door. A warning—not really a meaningfully helpful one from a safety perspective but more of an indication that the adults in charge weren't in the greatest headspace. This gist was this: "Stuyvesant is now more famous that anybody would like it to be. Please wear your ID badges at all times." Was this sign intended to imply that Stuyvesant was in danger of a terrorist attack? In the context of their other actions, that was certainly how the administration intended us to take it, so we did. Perhaps they were anticipating an attack by angry parents whose children had only gotten into Bronx Science? Or angry alumni disappointed with their selection of colleges? Surely Al-Qaeda had better targets to think about.

Or did they? In the climate of fear that had enveloped the nation by that point, we were ready to believe anything. Even that Al-Qaeda might have beef with the New York City Board of Education.

To me and many older students, the sign at the door felt heavy-handed but also reminiscent of the kind of hardheaded discipline that Principal Stanley Teitel had tried to instill when he first took the job in 1999. The Stuyvesant student body is smart and well behaved and enjoys a lot of freedom because of it, so even in the naive, pre-terror late nineties, students and teachers hadn't loved Principal Teitel's discipline-focused policy changes. Most of them, policies meant to police our whereabouts during free periods and that sort of thing, had ultimately failed. Now, however, he had the Bush administration on his side, not to mention a few willing generals in the school administration. One general apparently had access to a large-format printer and seemed eager to pass along any messaging that further validated our fear.

I carefully clipped my ID badge to my shirt with the small clasps they handed out and ducked inside, where the cool, air-conditioned air felt dry and smelled faintly burnt. I had the sensation of having to blow my nose for days after our return, which, along with my concerns about the smoky air meant I was spending a lot of time thinking about the simple act of breathing. Specifically, I felt as if I was not doing enough of it, but something instinctive in me seemed to be trying to limit the amount of Lower Manhattan air I inhaled.

AS WITH OUR FIRST day at Brooklyn Tech, a big back-to-school meeting was organized. This one was held in several shifts since our theater could not accommodate the entire school at once. I attended the last shift, right before dismissal, having already heard a number of concerning things about the agenda.

We began with the Pledge of Allegiance. After several weeks of practice with this tradition at Brooklyn Tech, I had perfected a strategy of sitting quietly during this recitation while making my point loudly. The country was in chaos, after all. Wars and invasions were already being broached by the Bush administration and were on everybody's mind—the White House was using language like "evil" to describe the enemy, threatening to unleash the "full wrath" of the United States military on this evil, and warning us that tackling this so-called evil would be an essentially never-ending obligation.[31] I remained unwilling to pledge allegiance to anything except a smooth college admissions process and clean air.

Principal Teitel, never one to let a meeting go by without instilling a little discomfort into the room, used this first meeting to make a few things clear. First, he enumerated our new post-terror policies. All of these policies were invariably designed to make the same point—that Stuyvesant was about to descend into fear-driven, undemocratic chaos, the very same chaos we had sworn to fight during the Pledge just minutes before.

Next up on the agenda, a reiteration of the warning on the sign earlier. Not wearing our IDs pinned to our clothing had become a punishable offense that would be met with the worst of all possible consequences—a mark on our permanent records and a call to our future colleges. At Stuyvesant, threatening to call colleges is tantamount to threatening jail time. Its power lies in the implication that Stuyvesant's administration can ruin your whole life if it wanted to, starting with a willingness to be complicit in your rejection from Yale, which will inevitably snowball into larger failures. Around this time the administration also disseminated an unsigned, almost parodyesque-sounding ID FAQ sheet that addressed this issue and reiterated their threat for the third time.

I still have two copies of this letter, one with a date marked on it indicating the day in late October that my mother called the school to complain about who on earth would send something of this nature to traumatized children. She found out who the author was—a computer science teacher, probably the same person terrorizing the school with the large-format printer. It was a Q&A with sample questions and mocking statements like:

"Ha! So, you admit that your ID card system could allow unauthorized people to get into the building. Someone could find a card or make one." These statement-like questions were followed by long-winded, sassy, uncopyedited answers like:

> Yes, it's true that the ID card requirement is not perfect but *it's better than nothing*. And the more that everyone complies the better it will be. We can't just sit around and wait for something to happen before we say, "Gee, I guess we should have been a little tighter on security. I hope the parents of those fourteen kids who died and thirty-seven who were injured understand about the sensitivity of Stuyvesant students to egregious burdens like wearing an ID card."

My favorite of the "questions" was "You fascist pigs with your Big Brother mentality are just trying to scare us. There's no real danger." The answer to that question began with:

> Are you for real? The biggest news event in the history of the world took place just a few blocks away from us and we were in the news frequently. There are bad people out there who believe that they will spend all eternity in heaven with seventy-two virgins if they can kill some of us while killing themselves. They really believe that.

Other "questions" suggested that students who missed the cutoff to test into Stuyvesant might want revenge. The whole thing was a real treat.

As the next priority on the assembly agenda, the principal confirmed that Stuyvesant was a potential target of a vague sort that he chose not to expand on. In the local news, bomb threats were all the rage, with journalists reporting on unmarked parcels and boxes in every corner of the city. As a result, despite its unlikeliness, we took this idea seriously. By that point we'd all heard about the rogue bomb threat the news reported from inside our school building on the eleventh itself, so anything was possible. I myself had already eyed numerous suspicious items all over the school, mostly unmanned backpacks. I'm sure I wasn't the only person who had to ask themselves, *How many unmanned backpacks did I used to see? How can I remember something I never thought to notice?*

Fourth on our meeting agenda was a new rule about minimizing our time outside. No going out to lunch, no sitting with friends on Chambers Street after school, no outside fun of any sort until the fires at Ground Zero stopped burning.

While the administration did buy into the numerous assurances from the Board of Education and the city that the school building was safe to inhabit in those early days, it was clear from their announcements that they still believed anything even an inch outside of the school building was dangerous. It seemed odd that this would not raise their suspicions about the air inside the building, since air is not beholden to any specific borders, but our principal had a soft spot for law and order and the assurances of officials, so we all just lived with the cognitive dissonance this caused.

A lot of outside/inside air conversation was also taking place outside the school among parents, politicians, and other officials. Word on the street was that the Board of Education had spent a whopping $1 million cleaning the building.[32] We were to treat that sum with respect. This was before the worst of the real estate boom and the complete devaluation of the $1 million sum to most New Yorkers, but in that circumstance, it still felt pithy. At the time of our meeting even the very seats we were sitting on—fabric auditorium seats in a carpeted theater—had not been cleaned or replaced. The carpet was later found to contain 250 times the legal limit of asbestos.[33] It wasn't swapped until the following August, when, according to local lore, a frustrated parent took a mat knife to a piece of the carpet, cut out a square, and had it tested. The Board of Education finally buckled when the results of that test made the newspaper and incoming parents begin to complain about holding the 2002 freshman orientation there. We, meanwhile, got to put on an entire year's worth of theater productions in that room before they tore out that toxic flooring. The upholstery, which was also contaminated, wasn't touched until 2014.[34] (Kids who didn't even remember 9/11 got the opportunity to be exposed to some leftover toxins. Living history, I guess?)

When the meeting was dismissed, the smell of smoke had already begun to infiltrate the hallways. This happened every afternoon. I walked past the northern windows on the way to my locker and stopped for a moment to watch the crane of a garbage barge, now moored next to the building to cart away Ground Zero debris, slowly move dusty wreckage from a line of cargo trucks onto a pile of rubble. Everything was metal and dust, and the noise alone nearly made me jump out of my skin. The barge, which, thanks to a waiver signed by Governor George Pataki[35] sat directly outside of our school's windows and air intake vents, was about to become a hot topic in Parents' Association and Board of Education circles, but for students it became a mesmerizing fact of life almost instantly. An actual toxic waste dump with new loads of pulverized everything arriving every few minutes, and it was literally a sidewalk's width from our windows. In those early days, not all of those windows were even closed.

I tried to hold my breath on the way back to the subway, but I couldn't.

AROUND 9:00 A.M. ON October 11, our third day back at the school, an alarm bell sounded. My already shaky nerves went into overdrive, and I was not the only one affected. Familiar looks of fear passed around my classroom. I was with Mr. Scotti, the same teacher I had been with on 9/11. I was again on the tenth floor. I was sitting across from the same person, watching a growing sense of urgency splash across his face.

There was one difference, of course. On September 11 no alarm bell had sounded, just the slightly shaky voice of the principal announcing that we would begin an evacuation after many assurances to the contrary. On

October 11, our teacher led us out of the unused doors on the south side of the building, doors we were not even allowed to enter through, doors that had been enveloped by the dust cloud on the eleventh and led to an area still closed off to the public. Apparently, the barge moored next door, that receptacle for the debris being removed from the World Trade Center site that was causing so much anxious conversation among parents, was not only polluting the air. It was also blocking our usual emergency escape route.

It was a confusing evacuation. Even those of us who were seniors and intimately familiar with Stuyvesant's myriad emergency escape routes had no idea where we were going. All we knew was that we were headed the wrong way as we exited the school and began to walk through Rockefeller Park in the direction of Ground Zero. In less chaotic times, students hung out in that park during lunch or after school—enjoying the expanse of grass with views of the river, the Statue of Liberty, and, for the curious, New Jersey. On that day, however, it was populated exclusively by National Guardsmen. They all had uniforms, huge dust masks that, at the time, I thought were World War II gas masks, and machine guns. We didn't even have our coats.

It may have only been a fire drill, but there was plenty of smoke rising above us as we fanned out along the edge of the park, sandwiched between our "burning" school and the burning rubble at Ground Zero. Stuck in a dead end. And if once wasn't enough, they sounded the alarm the next day too and repeated the whole ordeal. That second time, there was nothing to do but laugh.

As the days in the war zone passed, the administration committed further to a take-no-prisoners style of school governance, and the conversation about our safety became tense and public. It started with a quick turnaround in the position of the Parents' Association. In the first weeks after 9/11, over a series of private phone calls and exchanges, a powerful lobby of members, the PA's president included, had argued to the administration that a quick return of the students to Stuyvesant was necessary in order to maintain academic order. The initial plans to house both Brooklyn Tech and Stuyvesant at the same time in one Fort Greene building had seemed untenable, and parents flooded the chancellor's email box with demands that we return to Stuyvesant or use a split schedule so that the building wouldn't have to accommodate eight thousand students at one time. When they settled on the split schedule, the PA continued to press forward in asking for a speedy return to Stuy. According to *The Spectator*, Stuyvesant's school paper, PA president Christodoulou claimed that she was promised that by October 1 the Stuyvesant building would be under Stuyvesant's control:[36] "A twenty-four-hour cleanup crew is standing by; it will take between two and five days after the volunteers now using the building leave to clean it."[37] She told the paper, "It is very important to have the most continuity and the least disruption."[38]

Those same PA parents, Christodoulou included, found the smell of smoke inside the school alarming when we finally did reclaim the building. The poor air quality ignited feverish concerns about our safety. The administration responded with denials. At an uncharacteristically rowdy Parents' Association meeting on October 16, just after our return, Principal Teitel even asserted that if we were to leave the school for any period of time for health reasons, even if we made up the work at another high school, we would not be allowed to return. We were dealt the worst kind of choice, asked to decide between our present and our future, told we could have clean air or a good life, but not both.

Despite the amount of work I'd done just to get into Stuyvesant, the thought of leaving infiltrated my mind a lot in those early weeks. I was worried for my nerves, my asthma, my allergies, and my future health. The only thing that concerned me more than my health, however, was my college education. In the culture of Stuyvesant, that is neither an unusual priority nor an embarrassing thing to admit. Admission to a good college was the sole reason many of us stayed. Stuyvesant students are, in many ways, bred to base their self-worth on the caliber of college they get into. For some of us that pressure doesn't even come from our parents—I was considerably more obsessed with this than either of mine. So, we remained, silently cursing the unbending administration, knowing all the time that the school officials fully understood the choice they were imposing on us.

I heard rumors about a few students leaving—no one that I knew— but I did know one person who left because of the air quality. He wasn't a student; he was my math teacher. Rumors abounded as to where Mark Bodenheimer had gone and why, with some suggesting that he had been kicked out for complaining about Stuyvesant's conditions, others that he was willing to quit over it. The administration offered no comment. Then, the story broke in the press. He was the subject of a *New York Post* article on November 10, 2001, that began:

> A veteran Stuyvesant HS teacher has stayed away from his beloved school near Ground Zero for all but three days since it reopened Oct. 9, complaining foul air in and around the building has made him ill. "The air in the school smelled terrible. I'm refusing to go to Stuyvesant because it's a health problem for me," said thirty-year math instructor Mark Bodenheimer. Bodenheimer said he got a sore throat and headaches on the few days he did return to the school on the west end of Chambers Street, where it was once in the shadow of the World Trade Center.[39]

Mr. Bodenheimer ended up getting a decent deal. He was transferred to another competitive science school, Bronx Science. I learned this years later when he reached out to me, thanking me for my work related to his early concerns. Our math department had a very hard time filling his position. My class had a short-term substitute who stayed for months—longer, in fact, than the teacher whom they finally did find to replace him.

For the most part, however, a job at Stuyvesant, with its motivated and well-behaved students, is a pretty cushy gig for teachers. They, too, had reasons to stay, so most did.

DESPITE THEIR QUICK TURNAROUND on the school safety front, the PA learned the hard way in those first few weeks that it is easier to make a proactive decision than to undo one. With no reasonable way to move us out of the school building again, parents turned to the next battle—rallying for a more complete cleanup and a new location for the debris barge. After all, the EPA and Board of Education's assurances, even if you believed them, were undercut every time an uncovered truck full of debris drove past the school and dumped WTC dust right outside of our air intake and windows.

It was at that same rowdy Parents' Association meeting on October 16, attended by a massive crowd of over a thousand worried parents,[40] that my family learned that the conversation about school safety was not over. The meeting took place only a week after our return, and after forcing our parents through Stuyvesant's new patriotic ritual, the Pledge of Allegiance (my parents, true to form, abstained), the attendees were asked if their children were having health issues related to the environment at the school. The head of the PA told the school paper that about 20 percent of the crowd raised their hands—roughly two hundred parents.[41] The air quality consultant whom the PA had hired to investigate the safety of the building, Howard Bader, suggested the issues might be psychosomatic.[42]

A week and a half later my parents received a monster mailer from the PA's Environmental Health and Safety Committee. The report, dated October 26, stated that, despite the city's assurances, very few of the PA's original safety asks (the criteria that they believed would be met when they supported our return to Lower Manhattan) had been instituted.[43] The air ducts had not been examined for possible contamination, let alone cleaned. (There was, in fact, a lot of dust still lodged in them, and it wasn't cleared until the summer of 2002.) The outside air intake had not been shut off, and because of high CO_2 level readings inside the building, the city had actually increased the amount of contaminated outside air coming in around the time that students reoccupied the facility.[44] Parents had also been told that upgraded filters would be installed in the air system—they were not. What would be the point, anyway? The school's windows weren't even closed.

There was more, too. There was no certification from any public agency at any level of government showing that our building was safe to be reoccupied, and the footbridge students used to enter and exit the school was not being regularly cleaned despite the fact that it was covered in WTC dust and being recontaminated hundreds of times a day by the trucks carrying debris to the barge. There was no response from the city about whether they would move the debris barge to a less school-adjacent location. At the end of a ten-item list of air quality concerns, there were data concerns as well. As the PA wrote:

> We also learned that the EPA did not release to the public some monitoring results that appear to contradict or weaken its assertions of environmental safety. EPA data obtained by environmental activists using Freedom of Information Act requests appear to show more frequent and higher measurements of asbestos, heavy metals, PCBs, dioxin, benzene, and other toxins in and around the World Trade Center area than were previously acknowledged.[45]

It was our first indication that the EPA might have lied about the air quality downtown. The letter also included an updated report from Howard Bader, the consultant whose initial findings were the major reason the PA had supported the plan to return Stuyvesant to Lower Manhattan so quickly. Looking at data from the school in early October, he had basically said that there was no cause for concern, though at the time the main substance the Board of Education was testing for was asbestos, not the much longer list of chemicals later found in the downtown air.[46] He confirmed that he felt the building was safe in an interview with *The Spectator*, which printed an article about his findings entitled "An 'A' for Air Quality."[47]

By the time of the October report, students were already starting to experience health issues related to the WTC smoke just by living in town—a lot of New Yorkers endured headaches, chronic coughs, respiratory issues, nosebleeds, and other air-related health issues in those initial weeks of disaster recovery. On October 6 *The New York Times* reported that "many people who have moved back into downtown homes and offices are convinced that the air is unsafe, and they say they can produce their own data about the health risks: sore throats, tongue lesions, burning eyes and ears, and skin rashes."[48] One resident noted, "We feel physically sick when we stay there, sore throats, burning eyes, rashes."[49] By October 18, Stuyvesant's principal was reporting to parents that 57 students and 31 faculty members had already visited the nurse complaining of new symptoms, though he didn't address the rumors swirling that many more had given up on even seeing a nurse due to the long wait times and out-of-control lines.[50] A month later the *Times* reported of Stuyvesant that, "As many as eighty students and teachers have visited the school nurse with a range of ailments including headaches, itchy eyes, coughs, and even bloody noses."[51]

Either way, Bader's analysis changed after we'd been back in the building for a few weeks. His October 25 update confirmed that our school conditions were something to be concerned about, in part because the Board of Education had failed to take his recommended precautions. He reiterated the need for air filters and beefed up monitoring of the situation. He called the dust levels both inside and outside the school "unacceptable" and said they "represent a potential health concern."[52] A meeting to further address the air quality was set for my eighteenth birthday, November 13.

IN MOST PLACES, WATCHING a parent demonstrate outside your high school is not a part of the teenage experience, but during that school year many of us Stuyvesant students waved to our mothers and fathers as they held up signs questioning the safety of our school building on early post-9/11 mornings. The demonstrations got some coverage locally, but the challenges inherent in organizing for collective action were only exacerbated by the chaos of living in post-9/11 New York. It was difficult to get any traction. Other downtown community activists found the same thing—the news was hesitant to cover their work, the EPA denied negligence, and many in the city were desperate to move on.

It didn't help that beyond the usual community organizing obstacles—people have jobs and can't spend all day protesting in front of schools and calling public officials—Stuyvesant's parents faced some frustrating additional difficulties. There were language barriers and geographic barriers and the complications inherent in getting a bunch of incredibly detailed technical information to be understood by large numbers of people. Much of the student body wasn't from Lower Manhattan or anywhere close, so many Stuyvesant families had no frame of reference for just how bad things were downtown. For many parents there was no way to know they should be alarmed until months later, when the larger air quality issues, the ones that surrounded responders too, began to get more news coverage. In Chelsea, we could still smell the stench of WTC smoke when the wind blew the wrong way. Western Brooklyn was blanketed daily by thick clouds of WTC smoke. Yet, though *The Village Voice* noted that, "During the week that followed the attack, the acrid smell of burning plastic was so strong that residents far from Ground Zero mistakenly called in false alarms to fire departments in Queens, Nassau County, Brooklyn, and New Jersey,"[53] by October most of Queens, East Brooklyn, and Staten Island wasn't smelling burning chemicals in the air anymore. They were reeling in different ways, experiencing issues ranging from dealing with family losses to participating in the recovery efforts as responders to facing new and startling forms of racism and prejudice in the new world order. Their air wasn't opaque, though, so the Stuyvesant Parents living there couldn't have known the extent of what was going on downtown.

There was also the fact that many Stuyvesant kids were pretty excited to be returning to school because they were craving some normalcy. Their parents wanted to support this as best they could, much like the PA initially had wanted to. In February, *The New York Times* interviewed the father of one of my classmates from Queens who knew it was unsafe but wanted to respect his daughter's desire to stay.

> "My daughter would be very unhappy leaving, and I couldn't do it," he said. "But then I felt guilty for not doing it, so I'm caught in this quandary, removing her for health reasons or keeping her in because she loves the school."[54]

There were, of course, some people in denial too, including some of the Parents' Association's member base. This kind of bifurcation of concern within an affected community is common after a disaster—some people need to trust authority over all else to cope. Some need to think somebody else is the "real" victim in order to feel agency over their situation. To this day, some parents still won't hear of claims that the Board of Education acted irresponsibly and grow bizarrely angry when questioned. At this point these parents must defy established science in order to hang onto these beliefs. Many do anyway.

Eventually the very public consternation coming from the Parents' Association's leadership and the presence of widespread uncertainty about the safety conditions on the ground began to concern the school administration and Board of Education more broadly. They responded with increasingly strange behavior and more half-measures in the name of safety.

In early November Board of Education Deputy Chancellor David Klasfeld sent a letter to parents refuting the findings of the PA's latest environmental report and stating, "While there are occasional readings of moderately elevated levels of 'fine particulate matter,' which is undesirable, there is no evidence of the presence of an elevated level of any toxic substance at Stuyvesant."[55] That same month, however, the administration sent out a memo warning us not to drink out of the water fountains. Oddly enough, it was addressed to our parents, who were not in any danger of drinking school water. To be honest, most of us students were not in danger either—the school water was notoriously weird tasting and water fountains are germ factories anyway. Still, the memo floated around my house for months as my entire family grew increasingly appalled by its implication. Clearly, the administration knew the school building was unsafe, but was planning to protect us by sending out cryptic memos instead of engaging in any substantive action.

Soon after, men in biohazard suits began shuffling around the building, walking into classes with air meters, shaking their heads, and walking out. They set up air meters in the hallways as well, which made a hissing sound and did not appear to be controlled by anybody or checked in any way. The hissing became the soundtrack of the corridors between classes and after school. Our outside world had changed and now, inside, the hallways hissed. Word in the hallways was that the air meters were relatively useless—that they weren't designed to test for a lot of the chemicals and other toxins suspected to be in the air—but the charade calmed the nerves of those in the most denial and made the Board of Education look like it was doing something. What those meters continued to remind the rest of us of, however, was that even when we'd grown used to the smell of smoke, something bad was in the air.

When concerns about the air quality at Stuyvesant finally hit the national media, they yielded interesting results. In November a nursery in Orlando, Florida, donated a truckload of plants to the school so that at least something would be at work cleaning the air. They had not known whom to contact, so one day they simply showed up with a cargo truck and unloaded.[56] This was, in my opinion, the most touching gesture an outside entity made, but there were many others. Numerous schools donated murals and other artwork in solidarity, most of which got displayed along with our own mural attempts in random hallways, sometimes so deep into the building that you wouldn't see them until months after their arrival, when they'd pop up, deep in a back hallway on the seventh floor. Then, at some point in those early months, our head of maintenance brought me and some friends to the basement to show us the mother lode.

Stuyvesant's head of maintenance, a ubiquitous presence whose job description was vague and included nearly anything that had to be done, had been bristling about the number of donations the school was receiving for several weeks. We laughed about his annoyance. It was his responsibility to store and distribute these gifts, and most of us assumed this was an honor and he was just playing the grump. Finally, he grew sick of our teasing and decided to show a group of us why this generosity had become, in real, non-joking terms, a burden.

We took a set of unused stairs down to the basement. He produced a key that opened a steel door. We filed in, looked to our right, and were faced with the oddest thing. Next to the boiler room, in a storage space that was two to three times larger than my bedroom, was a pile two feet deep of notebooks, book bags, calendars, and other school supplies. It was, for an uninformed donor with access to said supplies and a notion that our school needed help, a thoughtful and appropriate gift. At the same time, it was a bizarre perception of our needs. As if somebody had thought: *They experienced a disaster. They must have lost all of their notebooks.*

In many cases, especially in war zones, this is entirely true. A school that burns down does, in fact, lose supplies, and in districts or countries where the needs run that basic, this gift would have been more than just a gesture, it would have meant real change. For Stuyvesant, however, it was a dilemma. Stuyvesant is well funded as public schools go.[57] It is a rare specimen of public school in that it has an endowment and textbooks and computer labs. The students have notebooks. They have book bags. Nobody had lost any pencils in the disaster.

The gifts sat in a pile in the basement, untouched, until somebody finally donated them to another school. On the day we went downstairs, however, I took a notebook just to show that their gesture of generosity hadn't gone totally unnoticed. It was still sitting on my shelf, empty, when I left for college the next year. I brought it with me and used it in my first semester, a small, secret piece of commemorative disaster paraphernalia for when I felt nervous and out of place among my college's more functional, less traumatized students.

The real issue was that, for us students in the moment, our problems were intangible. They could not be addressed with stuff. They were memories and smells and tastes. They were the sudden moment you'd notice the acrid smell of the air again after growing accustomed to it. The knowledge that you'd been sitting in that air for hours. The churning worry that if you'd been oblivious to that smell, you were probably missing other hazards too. If anything, we probably needed therapy, but even that donated resource was going unused.

There was tremendous pressure to act casual about everything unless you needed therapy, and if you did then it was okay to fall apart in a dramatic manner. For my part, I felt stuck in some middle level of neurosis that, mixed with my lack of experience with therapy, general dislike of touchy-feely things, and memory of that September 12 phone call with my aunt and uncle, led me to believe I could take care of my problems myself. It was probably clear to most outsiders that, in reality, I could not. Meanwhile, rumor had it that the teachers' therapist was offering participants cake while the student therapy sessions were snack-free. I might have shown up for some cake.

Therapy or no therapy, my heightened level of distraction bothered me immensely. There were butterflies in my stomach all day, every day—those never went away. One shout by an unsuspecting teenager would cause me to drop things, whip around without looking, and employ other hasty movements that put all of the inanimate objects in my vicinity in danger. I nervously jumped at every sound of an airplane's descent and every crash from the truckloads of debris being dropped off at the barge. I once even tried complaining to my congressman that they, the big "they," were rerouting flights to descend over the Hudson River just to make us crazy. In retrospect that's a very silly thing to tell your congressman, but, notably, he told me I was not the only person who had raised that issue with him.

Quiet, of course, was not any easier for me. Before 9/11, noise was my refuge from the overwhelming influx of distracting thoughts I experience if left to my own devices. A lot of New Yorkers experience this—neutral in the city is pretty noisy, so "normal" and, by extension, calm, is pretty loud. When I was a freshman, several construction sites had popped up around Stuyvesant, running their pile drivers all day to find bedrock below the landfill they were building on. One science class determined that the constant shaking of the building these pile drivers caused was equivalent to a permanent 3.0 magnitude earthquake, but that still didn't consider the steady sound of metal hitting metal. It had been loud and theoretically disruptive, but, somehow, it had filtered out my nonacademic thoughts. Helped me think clearly. The crane on the debris barge and the passing trucks were making a rhythmic sound, but it was having the opposite effect. The type of noise did not matter. Happy noises, sad noises, alarming noises, expected noises—all of them made me jump. And then quiet; the quiet was the worst part because when I was left with no noise, my head created the noises. Those sounds were less startling but always more gruesome.

CHAPTER 5

DEBRIS

In January, the fires at Ground Zero finally burned out. Enough of the debris had been cleared by then that the intersection at Greenwich Street became, once again, unremarkable. Our lunch privileges resumed, so we were allowed to wander the neighborhood in search of food. My favorite pizza place reopened.

As the cleanup efforts continued, we settled into an anxious routine. Sites of destruction were so normalized that I could finally watch the barge operations without thinking about how many bodies were in the rubble. Every once in a while, however, we'd be reminded that we were living in an extraordinary time. On one cold morning, and I don't remember when, we walked up to the school to find that the mangled remains of the globe statue that had sat between the Twin Towers was parked in front of our school. I kept waiting for somebody to note how insanely thoughtless it was to leave that statue there at 8:45 a.m. on a school day so that thousands of traumatized students would have to walk by it, but nobody said a word.

Beyond Chambers Street, change continued to churn. New Yorkers said goodbye to the city's own Principal Teitel, New York's chaotic law-and-order-loving mayor Rudy Giuliani, who spent his lame duck session riding a wave of national glory. There was brief talk of letting him serve a third term as mayor to help New York heal. At my house, we blamed that talk on transplants—non-native New Yorkers, that naive breed. Luckily, enough of us remembered how much we'd hated Rudy on September 10, 2001. (Note to future mayors: Never *ever* try to criminalize jaywalking.)

In the final few months of his term, Giuliani's tendency toward bizarre, erratic, and sometimes corrupt behavior had been on full display. My parents and I privately joked about how, in a fit of peak corrupt, ill-conceived Giuliani-ness, "America's Mayor" had moved the Office of Emergency Management (OEM), the city's emergency response head-quarters, into the World Trade Center itself, rendering it largely useless during and after the attacks.[58] *The Village Voice* reported: "Sam Caspersen, one of the principal authors of the 9/11 Commission's chapter on the city's response, says that 'nothing was happening at OEM' during the 102 minutes of the attack that had any direct impact on the city's 'rescue/ evacuation operation.'" The article also notes that "the OEM had no high-rise plan—its emergency-management trainers weren't even assigned to prepare for the one attack that had already occurred, and the one most likely to recur."[59] This disclosure is especially wild because, even before 2001, any random New Yorker would have told you that the World Trade Center was the city's most likely terrorist target, and according to the Giuliani administration's (slightly revisionist) history of the OEM, it had only been established in the first place because the Twin Towers had been bombed before.[60] Rumor at the time was that Giuliani's choice to build the command center at the World Trade Center was linked to an affair he was having.

The decision to place the bunker at the WTC site was actually linked to a Republican developer connected to the mayor, but Giuliani's fingerprints were everywhere; the bulletproof office Giuliani kept there—which he fre-quented with his illicit love Judith Nathan—had monogrammed towels, a humidifier for cigars, and a private elevator.[61] In what was my favorite story of the era, his affair with Nathan resulted in his being kicked out of Gracie

Mansion, the mayoral housing, by his ex-wife, and moving into the spare room of a gay couple who owned a bunch of car dealerships in Queens as well as a small shih tzu named Bonnie.[62] The story that he'd been kicked out of Gracie Mansion broke on September 2, 2001, just over a week before the World Trade Center attacks, and is key context for anybody looking to understand the political environment that September 11 altered. Either way, there's a reason New Yorkers didn't go for his third-term bid.

AT THE NATIONAL LEVEL, the political environment was less salacious but more concerning. The conversation about when and where to go to war began within a few weeks of 9/11. Congress passed a use-of-force authorization in late September 2001, which allowed:

> That the President is authorized to use all necessary and appropriate force against those nations, organizations, or persons he determines planned, authorized, committed, or aided the terrorist attacks that occurred on September 11, 2001, or harbored such organizations or persons, in order to prevent any future acts of international terrorism against the United States by such nations, organizations or persons.[63]

With this authorization the United States launched a military operation in Afghanistan,[64] but the war talk hit a fever pitch in late fall when Bush uttered the now infamous words: "You're either with us or against us in the fight against terror."[65] Those words instantly become the shorthand for the behavior we were all supposed to exhibit, part of an organizing framework that was internalized and recapitulated by the press to the point that it defined the political and cultural climate.[66] Most frustrating was that the "us versus them" dialogue seemed intent on using our losses in New York to justify violence somewhere—anywhere—else.

Soon, after information about Bush's interest in Iraq began to leak in late winter, the president began to officially build a case against Saddam Hussein's oil-rich nation. Bush first uttered the words the "axis of evil," to classify nations that harbored, financed, and aided terrorists—namely Iran, North Korea, and Iraq—in his January 2002 State of the Union address.[67] It was the first time he connected Iraq to weapons of mass destruction, saying of the axis of evil nations, "By seeking weapons of mass destruction, these regimes pose a grave and growing danger."[68]

By drawing the explicit connection between Iraq, WMDs, and terrorism, verbalizing a doctrine rooted in preemptive action, and asserting that the war on terror had only just begun,[69] Bush laid the groundwork on which he would carefully build a case for war in Iraq.[70] Meanwhile, the dust and debris sitting in Stuyvesant's ventilation system stayed put. Our symbolic value was more important than our actual value, apparently. We diligently carried on, no longer able to smell the toxic stew in the air but all the while aware it was there.

From my high school perch, the Iraq war dialogue was incredibly frustrating and, in many ways, heartbreaking. Not because I was a great lover of Iraqi dictators, but because I was a great lover of basic logic.

There are layers to the kinds of heartbreak you feel if you live through a traumatic event that has the visibility of 9/11. There's the day itself. There's the long process of coming to terms with how much change it has caused in your daily life—an event like 9/11 even changes your outlook on the things that didn't change. Once safe places don't look safe anymore. Once unremarkable noises don't feel unremarkable. The crowded city landscape, the density of which once brought comfort, suddenly looks like it's teeming with potential dangers. It was not unlike in the early months of the COVID-19 pandemic, when invisible virus particles suddenly made even the empty air between us seem potentially deadly. Most Americans can now relate to this layer of heartbreak. Going to a concert and getting on an airplane changed after 9/11, and, after 2020, we'll probably never even return to that version of "normal."

Then there is the fact that everybody on Earth believes they personally experienced 9/11. On some level they did, but not everybody viscerally experienced the smell of burning debris, and most people don't live with health concerns because of it. That's a gap you can never properly articulate or bridge even with your closest friends and family.

And then, finally, there's the fact that mass violence has political consequences, always, and those consequences feel very personal when you are the symbol being used to justify them.

FROM MY ADULT PERCH, I can now see that part of what makes mass violence so frustrating is that people who are left very afraid in the aftermath of an act of violence do weird and illogical things. A lot of powerful people, as it turns out, do not handle their fear all that productively. Not that I do. My instinctive response to fear is avoidance, or, if there's something I absolutely have to face, negotiation. At worst, I filibuster. I never think to throw a punch. On a cellular level, the logic of responding to violence with more violence has never made sense to me. It only heightens my fear and worsens my experience. Still, I could see some inherent logic in the conversation around sending troops to Afghanistan, the place that had enabled an attack on us, even if it wasn't how I would have personally directed the response. Iraq was a different story.

On a personal level, I felt a tremendous sense of guilt and responsibility for allowing this dialogue about avenging our losses to happen, but I also had no channels through which to meaningfully resist it. There is no way to disengage from the cycle of political violence that gets set into motion after an event like 9/11. That was a lesson I was young and optimistic enough not to already know and wasn't prepared to learn with such force.

The fact that nobody seemed to care about the dilemma they'd created for us teenagers—the feeling of responsibility and helplessness that era engendered—was the rudest awakening of the whole experience. I had—and still have—a lot of anger about what happened to me, but there was also a lot of grief. That particular grief—the grief that grew out of losing control of my narrative and being used as symbol—is one that still pulls at me. It's an underlying tension of every interaction I've had about 9/11 and the community's health since. So many people who were eager to use me and my classmates to justify unnecessary violence just don't seem to care about the cost of that violence on us or, frankly, the people we inflicted it on. That dissonance, which they so easily live with, breaks my heart.

At the time, however, only a few months clear of 9/11, I could only articulate the loneliness that came with being a symbol. Even inside Stuyvesant everybody experienced the tension in the air differently, and it somehow became more isolating the more we discussed it. There were anti-war campaigners, of course, but there were also students arguing that we had to do *something*. Many New Yorkers were vocally frustrated by the Iraq discussion, but not *all* of them were. And some of them began to turn their fear into other kinds of violence, including hate crimes and acts of aggression that imperiled the safety of good friends, many of whom were struggling with the same larger questions. By September 17, 2001, the Council on American-Islamic Relations was already reporting a notable uptick in reports of harassment and abuse, getting more than three hundred calls in the three days following September 11.[71] Sikhs, Hindus, and other South Asian communities were all targeted as well, and the tentacles of this danger stretched longer than what the statistics could ever demonstrate. Numbers don't account for the layer of fear this created for New Yorkers of South Asian descent and the extra preventative measures they had to begin taking to stay safe. Friends were told they couldn't travel the city as freely as they once had, not because of terrorism, but for fear of harassment. The mother of my close friend Indrina, the same friend who called me on 9/11 and offered up her home in Queens as a safe harbor, was told on September 11 by a policeman neighbor that she should avoid wearing her regular Indian clothes outside of the house for her safety.

I turned eighteen in November 2001, so 9/11 closed a chapter on my childhood in ways that were literal as well. Because of our age, the other war-related worry that circled around my classmates and me was whether there would be a draft. I'd never once thought about the Selective Service System—the military draft list that, at the time, only boys had to sign up for if they wanted to be able to get college loans and other services. Amid the growing drumbeat of war—a first major conflict of our generation—there was real reason to worry we might be drafted to fight in some part (and potentially not the correct part) of the Middle East. As if that anxiety was something a bunch of scared teenagers in the middle of the WTC recovery effort needed on their plate.

Luckily for me, the Selective Service System was only for men. I'd never been so thrilled to be on the losing end of the patriarchy. But, as my boomer parents fretted, I also knew I didn't want to be part of a Vietnam generation.

THOUGH IT WASN'T AS splashy as a war, air quality discussions did continue, largely unreported in national media, on the ground in the neighborhoods around us and between our Parents' Association and the Board of Education. In January and February a series of letters and angry memos were fired back and forth between the Parents' Association and the school administration. On January 31 the Parents' Association Board voted to pursue possible legal action against the city. On February 4 an update was sent to parents with a report from the PA Health and Environmental Safety Committee. It listed a litany of remaining concerns about the school ventilation system, the barge operating next door, and the lack of adequate environmental testing.[72] The committee's findings included that the air system, which was the building's only air intake route since the windows had to be closed to prevent WTC dust from entering, had still not been cleaned.[73] The fancy filters that would have prevented dangerous chemicals from entering the building had still not been installed and could not be because the air system would have to be retrofitted for them.[74] Air quality measures taken inside the building were showing levels of particulate matter that exceeded EPA guidelines for children.[75] And, of course, there was still the debris barge adjacent to the school, at which the PA had measured levels of particulate matter in the air and found that they were, on many days, higher than at Ground Zero itself.[76] The report also mentioned an onslaught of new health issues at the school, stating:

> Many parents report that their children have experienced unusual rashes, nosebleeds, coughing attacks, and chronic sinus and respiratory problems, including new onset asthma and chemical bronchitis.[77]

The letter also noted that, despite Principal Teitel's ban on their return, eleven students had left due to health problems, as had several staff members beyond Mr. Bodenheimer. Like students, staff and custodians were also getting sick with nosebleeds, rashes, sinus issues, bronchitis, and other respiratory illnesses. (In late April the National Institute for Occupational Safety and Health, NIOSH, confirmed as much, releasing a report that noted that after October 9, 50 to 60 percent of the Stuyvesant staff had reported respiratory symptoms, the majority of which were new onset.[78]) The letter also mentioned that the teacher's union had filed a grievance and that a special PA general meeting would be held on February 13.[79]

Deputy Chancellor of the Board of Education David Klasfeld responded to the February 4 report in a February 7 letter to the school community in which he noted his "grave disappointment with a recent communication sent to you from the Stuyvesant Parents' Association's Environmental Health and Safety Committee." His letter included a point-by-point rebuttal of the PA's letter, but many of the passages were simply explanations for why the city couldn't address the PA's demands or shouldn't need to. Of the calls for better air filtration, he stated:

Stuyvesant's HVAC system, which is part of a superior, $200 million facility, is only ten years old (far from old when looking at the average age of other school buildings in New York City) and does provide for a more than adequate internal air environment for the school.[80]

He called the air quality at Stuyvesant "excellent" multiple times and dismissed the alarming health reports as "anecdotal" before ending with an upbeat promise that, "The Board of Education has never stopped working toward providing the Stuyvesant Community with the tools to make the school a safe and secure learning environment."[81] The letter, passages of which, to me, feel like they are gaslighting the reader, only further escalated the situation. The PA's Environmental Health and Safety Committee followed up by issuing a point-by-point rebuttal of his point-by-point rebuttal—a single-spaced four-page report with citations of supporting medical research.[82]

To add further chaos, a subgroup of angry PA board dissenters passed out their own letter during the back and forth, explaining that they were opposed to the PA's suing the city. Their reasons included the confounding excuse that the conversation was bringing "negative attention to Stuyvesant at a time when families across the city are deciding where to send their children to high school."[83] They agreed with Klasfeld that there was "no convincing data" that the school was dangerous anymore and felt that while they supported moving the debris barge, they also understood that the city had no ability to do that, so, they asked, why bother continually highlighting it. They ended the letter by noting that there "is no absolute safety" in life. The letter, with passages set in all caps, reads as if its writers are incredibly angry but also incredibly scared. Among the PA members, the dissenters did not fall along predictable lines. While my parents fretted about my breathing, which had gotten measurably worse in the months since our return, the mother of one of my oldest friends was a cosigner on the opposition letter. Conversations among students began to reflect this rift.

All parties packed into the same room for the February 13 special PA meeting, which was attended by representatives from the city, the dissenting board members, and some parents who hadn't been party to any of these ongoing conversations. It was at this meeting where many casual PA members, those like my parents who were not involved in the committees, learned more about the extent of the city's failings and the PA Environmental Health Committee's concerns. Still, aside from the student and teacher departures, most of what my parents learned at that meeting could be summarized as *nothing has meaningfully changed since October*. The school and the city had taken very few, if any, steps in response to the concerns the PA was raising, even as their concerns continued to mount.

The February notices are angry and thorough, but also show clear indications that battle fatigue had started to set in. That's not surprising—the victories the PA did win often dissipated as if by magic. In the late winter parents had won a small battle in the war against the debris barge, requesting that the contents of the trucks passing daily by our school be hosed down (as had been initially promised) so dust wouldn't trail off behind the trucks and land all over the neighborhood. Visible dust covered everything outside by this point, not just because of the initial dust cloud, but because the cleanup effort was peppering the area with new dust every day. Unfortunately, they won this battle just before the weather made it a moot point. Once the temperatures dipped below freezing, hosing the trucks down became an impossibility.[84]

On the heels of the February 13 meeting, the city decided to send another mailing, this time enclosing a letter from the chair of the Department of Community and Preventative Medicine at Mount Sinai Hospital. His letter, dated February 20, claimed that the air was fine—"Now that the fires are out, I believe on the basis of my review of the air data that the quality of the outdoor air around the World Trade Center is not appreciably different from that in many areas of New York City,"[85]—and that he'd advise against revising the air system at Stuyvesant now because it would churn up more hazards than it would prevent "through the inevitable creation of construction dust."[86] Essentially, they had stalled so long that fixing the problem would be more dangerous than letting it go. Years later a custodial staff member showed me pictures from the great vent cleaning project of the summer of 2002. In the photos, the vents are lodged with a several-inches-deep layer of black dust. At a hearing organized by the EPA's ombudsman on February 27, the New York City Schools chancellor Howard Levy was asked whether he could show any evidence that the data proving the downtown schools were being recontaminated by WTC dust daily was *not* true. He could not.[87]

Klasfeld and the dissenting parents were forced to eat their words within a couple of months anyway. Among the missives firing back and forth in February was a letter from the PA's air quality consultant Howard Bader, dated February 7, in which he notes that new samples show that the school has dangerously elevated lead levels.[88] In June, just before the end of the school year, the Board of Education released its own data, based on samples taken back in April, that showed the same elevated levels.[89] Two things were clear: first, that these findings became the impetus for their eventual cleanup of the school's air system that summer; second, the Board of Education ignored the data for months before it finally acted.

Regardless of what the city was saying, my pulmonologist had concerns. I've been asthmatic since childhood, but at the beginning of high school I had finally found a treatment program that worked. It changed my life. I even joined the cross-country team, which had been so wildly outside my capabilities the year before that I didn't even worry that I was terrible. I loved everything about being on that team, from the long train trips we took uptown to do our runs, all gossip-filled and energetic, to the pastries we'd buy on the way home, to the unlikely friendships it allowed for with people I'd never have otherwise crossed paths with. The cross-country world was a nice community too. Once, during a race, a competitor from another team noticed me having asthma issues on a big hill and literally took my hand to pull me up the slope with her. When we got to the top she asked, "You okay?" and waited for me to nod before continuing on her way.

9/11 was a major setback to my treatment success, and effectively ended my cross-country career. My doctor, Dr. Ting, was a resident of the area around Stuyvesant himself, so he knew what the quality of the air was when we returned and in the time that had passed since. He was also, notably, a Stuyvesant alum. When I went to see him, he told me, "Look, I don't know what to tell you. You shouldn't be down there, but I know you can't leave Stuyvesant in your senior year." Even outside of Mr. Teitel's insistence that students could not leave and graduate with a Stuyvesant diploma, my doctor, a Stuyvesant graduate himself who had attended college and medical school and been in the workforce for years, inherently understood I could not leave. Instead, my parents watched the air quality discussion with a growing feeling of powerlessness. None of us knew what to do with Dr. Ting's advice other than not think too hard about it. We did continue to attend protests outside the school. After one protest requesting the city move the debris barge, we even wound up pictured in the *New York Daily News*.

BY MARCH, EVERY LOWER Manhattan school had returned students to the immediate area around Ground Zero and most of the neighborhood's residents were back in their homes.

The six-month anniversary of the attacks rolled around. That week the nation was desperately taking stock of the whirlwind we'd gone though, placing all of its attention on a controversial documentary that was filmed at the World Trade Center on September 11 and aired the evening of March 10 on CBS. The project, called simply *9/11*, was the work of Jules and Gédéon Naudet, two French brothers who happened to be documenting a downtown fire department's activities when the World Trade Center call came in. They were the only professional crew to get a shot of the first plane hitting the towers, and as they rushed inside the lobby of the North

Tower and watched a chaotic evacuation unfold as the South Tower fell, they did a very human thing: they started cursing. CBS elected to air the documentary unedited and, notably, unbleeped, which only heightened the buzz around the project.

By March 2002 I had watched the attacks from many angles on television. The footage was on repeat for months on every channel. I felt immune to it. Plus, the buzz around the documentary was inescapable, so while I wasn't exactly eager to watch it, curiosity got the better of me. I hit my permanent limit for watching 9/11 videos that night. The documentary was viscerally terrifying for me in a way that no other film about this event has ever been. It wasn't the fact that we weren't very removed from the experience yet, nor the fact that they captured shots of the planes flying or the explosions. It was the lobby footage.

The huge scale of the Twin Towers meant that footage of the attacks was almost always shot from very far away. Even the pictures of people running that day generally include the huge scale of the danger behind them. People appear tiny in those photos. None of the iconic news shots of 9/11 include much that reflects on the experience of evacuating from inside an unknown danger. The footage is of the danger itself—two large towers in flames. As I evacuated, I had a full view of the attack going down, so while I had myriad reasons to be concerned on that day between the potential for further attacks and not really understanding the physics of how a large building collapses, I knew exactly what I was running from. I could see the borders of the disaster.

The documentary that aired on the six-month anniversary showed us 9/11 from the inside of the towers, where the danger was much more amorphous. The filmmakers spend a lot of time on the ground in places where they can't really see what's going on because the fires are far above them. There is wreckage outside, but the scale of the crisis is not visible to any of the people rushing by. The lobby is both chaotic and disturbingly quiet in the shots—the lights are out, people wander aimlessly. They are scared, but nobody has any idea just how scared to be, where the danger is, or how to get to safety. After all, they can't really see where danger ends and safety begins.

I knew the lobbies of the World Trade Center well. My friends and I had spent hours hanging out there—the mall below was a perfect mix of browsing opportunities and subway accessibility. Around the time of the attacks I didn't think much about losing that hangout, or any hangout for that matter, because it seemed like nobody would ever hang out ever again anyway. (What kind of insane person would elect to reenter a terrorist target with people and just . . . sit there?) But watching confusion and fear overtake the faceless mob of suit-people I used to see in those lobbies was alarming. Witnessing their indecision about which direction would be safe because they, unlike me, could not see the borders of the disaster, was painful. It was the only film where I watched a familiar, human-scale hangout get destroyed without the distraction of watching a fireball engulf a larger-than-life icon. I did not like the view.

TECHNICALLY THE RECOVERY OPERATIONS ended on May 30, 2002,[90] though the cleanup efforts continued in smaller ways until long after.[91] During a commemorative ceremony that day, a solemn parade passed by the school midday, and students distractedly rushed to windows to watch as bagpipes made their way up the West Side Highway. Then, like now, I couldn't handle all the solemnity around 9/11. It made the trauma of the day too present and tangible. I briefly caught sight of the parade heading by but immediately walked away from the windows when the bagpipes started playing. There is nothing more solemn than bagpipes. There is also nothing first responders love more than a parade or ceremony with bagpipes. It's an area where we absolutely do not see eye to eye.

By that May, a lot of the changes around us were no longer notable. Men in orange suits shuffled in and out of our classes monitoring the air quality, and that seemed normal. The school was still draped in murals sent by other schools, but they started to look like a regular part of the scenery. Every plane that flew overhead made the entire student body jump, but since it was every single plane and every single person it, too, became a part of life.

The school's drama program also returned. The season began with a unique project—at the beginning of the spring semester Annie Thoms, the same young English teacher who had taken over my SSR at Brooklyn Tech at the last minute, organized a play in the style of an Anna Deavere Smith, a renowned dramatist who is known for a distinct style of documentary theater based off of interviews with real people. Student participants interviewed members of the Stuyvesant community about their experiences on and after 9/11, then performed monologue versions of the interviews in character. It was a controversial project at the time. A lot of people thought it was too soon. I was among them. Maybe it was, though I did run the lighting grid for the production (nerd!). The monologues were hard to listen to, and as somebody practicing as much avoidance as humanly possible, I strained to sit through them at every rehearsal and performance.

In retrospect that play, called *with their eyes: September 11th—The View From a High School at Ground Zero*, was probably the most successful thing the Stuyvesant Theater has ever produced. It was published as a book and now other schools perform it every year. It's one of the few collections of 9/11 stories that include legitimate moments of levity—it's solemn but relatable. While it felt too soon to me at the time, the interviews were done quickly enough that the memories the play describes are fresh. They hadn't been confused or absorbed by the larger narrative. It was very easy to project the stories we all heard ad nauseam onto our personal 9/11 experience—I probably have done it many times in these pages without realizing it. *with their eyes* documents life before we had a chance to do that.

Spring at Stuyvesant also brought about the biggest annual theater event of the year—SING! A number of New York City schools have this tradition; essentially a competition in which each class puts on a student produced, written, acted, danced, and sung musical and competes in front of an alumni judging panel. Since the panel is all alumni, the results are usually more tradition than anything else. Seniors win. Juniors come in second. Soph-frosh, which is a combined sophomore and freshman class show, usually loses. When there are upsets it is very big news. That year our SING! show (the exclamation point is a vital part of the word) was set in a bowling alley in the eighties. The show was silly, as every SING! production is, but it was the first thing that felt truly normal about the year. Everybody remembers their senior SING! fondly, and I remember ours like it was a cup of hot cocoa. It was hard work, as always, but it was also easy and familiar and comforting to be a part of. It was a brief reprieve, a chance to visit in on childhood for a few hours a day. A chance to pretend we lived in a different era.

NOBODY WOULD HAVE FRAMED it this way at the time, but there were some perks to being part of the nation's premiere high-profile disaster, too. I learned in January that I'd gotten into Vassar College early and was able to sit around smugly when college acceptance letters arrived that spring, but students, by and large, got into all of their first choice colleges. Almost everybody wrote their essays about 9/11, and the sympathy vote was real.

Then there was the fact that Bill Clinton spoke at my high school graduation. Clinton's legacy is a little more complicated now, but at that time there was truly nobody bigger to dream for as a commencement speaker. Public high schools in New York City did not usually get ex-presidents to speak at graduation, and there was nobody in more demand than Clinton himself. Our graduation took place at Lincoln Center, and despite the size of Avery Fisher Hall, it was a hot ticket—I wasn't even able to score seats for my grandparents.

I like to tell people that graduation was fun and Clinton's speech was great, but in all honesty I don't remember much about the ceremony. The only truly memorable moment for me was a bizarre exchange I had during the rehearsal in which the smaller, more imperceptible life changes that had occurred in the last year caught up with me. I was lined up along the wall in a hallway at Avery Fisher Hall, standing with my homeroom and waiting to practice walking in. While we waited and joked around about how hard it is to walk in straight lines, my math teacher—I'd hesitantly elected to take the second semester of calculus after my first semester teacher left due to health concerns—saw me waiting. Without thinking, he blurted out, "Oh good, you're graduating."

This teacher was a soft-spoken guy, generally understood to be nice, but even the people standing around me looked at him quizzically. He realized, too late, how his comment had sounded. He wandered off. I, meanwhile, was left in a state of shock about what I must have been projecting in his class. What kind of student he thought I was. He was somebody I had never taken a class with before 9/11—he only knew me after. Apparently my "after" self was not somebody I recognized, because I am somebody who is, at the most basic, most intrinsic level, a very good student. In the context of Stuyvesant I knew I wasn't *the best*—you have to be nearly perfect to be notable at Stuy—but, still, my entire identity was linked to being a high achiever. My grades in every other subject were fine, but his comment was, I think, a testament to how unconvincingly I was holding it together at that time.

I got a B in that math class, by the way. That's only a failure by Stuyvesant standards (and only a Stuyvesant student would still remember this fact twenty years later).

Though by graduation day most of life had returned to some degree of normalcy, there was one thing that reminded us daily that life was never going to be the same—the administration's continuing insistence on doing the Pledge of Allegiance. We did it every morning, and we did it at that graduation ceremony too. That change was forever—I recently found out that they still do the Pledge at Stuyvesant every day. Every few years the topic makes an appearance in the school paper. Some people don't say the Pledge. Some people do. By now nobody asks why the tradition started.

CHAPTER 6

BEGINNINGS OF
MEMORIES

College is a difficult adjustment for everybody. There are new rooms, new people, long linoleum tables filled with Aramark™ food and non–New Yorkers who think it's funny you don't know anything about cars. They'll tell you that you talk too fast, that you develop an accent on the phone with your parents—which you've never been told before, and how dramatic an accent can it be if nobody has ever mentioned it before? They'll recount the deb (debutante) balls they went to back home, which don't even sound like a real thing. They'll do all of this while eating light, barely visible salads that keep their Freshman Fifteen at bay as you slowly balloon, deep in the grasps of the Freshman Thirty. They'll top off their meals with Froyo, but they'll get it without toppings and throw it out halfway through while you dig the candy out of your own.

Moving away from home is anxious work. Recurrent nightmares don't help. I was having them regularly. Stuy friends who had gone to college elsewhere were having them as well, but we never spoke about it then. It was years before I found out how common this was. Instead we all woke up alone, startled to see a near-stranger sleeping in the bed next to ours and an unfamiliar (but unharmed) room surrounding us.

For me, the nightmares were always about the Empire State Building, and the event that inspired them was pretty clear from the content. A plane would fly into the top of the tower (a little on the nose), or the spire would catch fire, or I'd be running down an endless series of stairwells. When there were thunderstorms, which felt extreme already because they were so much louder and brighter in my Hudson Valley dorm room than they had been in Manhattan, the thunder and lightning would find their way into the dream. Cracks of thunder would become the sounds of metal or machinery hitting the building. At the flashes of lightning, I'd wake up, sleepily checking my surroundings to verify whether something terrible was going on. I remember the dreams so well because they usually woke me up. This was, of course, before school shootings became a weekly occurrence. At least when I woke up, I had the comfort of knowing that nobody in their right mind would actually attack Vassar's campus. I was, by design, living somewhere random enough to be safer than home. Kids these days, attending school in an era of regular, localized, mass violence, probably do not have that assurance when a nightmare wakes them in their first weeks of college.

EVEN WHEN I WAS awake, Poughkeepsie, New York, didn't offer me much. Despite the hilarious name and Hudson Valley setting, it felt like it had more in common with postindustrial Detroit than the neighboring vacation enclave of Rhinebeck. I made friends in my first weeks and spent the weekends proudly showing them my hometown instead of staying on campus. I convinced myself that being from New York was my most interesting quality, not because of 9/11 but because of television. Because it was creative and seedy and still somehow wealthy and cultured. As I toured out-of-towners around, I conveniently left out the scary parts, the sites of destruction. We'd sit in fancy coffee shops, then get fries on St. Mark's Place. I'd point out the building I lived in as a child there but leave out the parts about the murders and cannibals (the East Village in the eighties was a wild place), the black market on the corner, the very curious air-shaft mosquito problem that plagued our apartment. I'd cover my anxious tics, my tendency to jump at the slightest noise, by continually moving, skipping, always talking, laughing, filling every silence. I pretended to be into photography so we could wander the city as tourists, letting it reflect *Sex and the City*'s New York back to us instead of my own.

As I basked in Carrie Bradshaw's New York, fine-tuning my approach afterward by watching the series on the floor of my dorm's hallway, the drumbeat of war continued, still pushing a heavy dose of guilt and frustration at me. By the fall of 2002 the bombing of Iraq was already old news—it had begun back in June,[92] just as my senior year of high school wrapped up and I headed into a summer of pre-adult panic and obsessive dorm room shopping. In late August, as I was packing up to head out into the world on my own for the first time, Dick Cheney had given a speech in which he said, "there is no doubt that Saddam Hussein now has weapons of mass destruction; there is no doubt he is amassing them to use against our friends . . . and against us."[93] In mid-September, as school began and I met my roommate and new classmates for the first time, George Bush made a now infamous speech before the UN in which he spoke in stark, confident terms about Iraq's supposed weapons arsenal and the imminent threat it posed:

> The history, the logic, and the facts lead to one conclusion: Saddam
> Hussein's regime is a grave and gathering danger. To suggest otherwise
> is to hope against the evidence. To assume this regime's good faith is to
> bet the lives of millions and the peace of the world in a reckless gamble,
> and this is a risk we must not take.[94]

Just a couple of weeks into my school year at Vassar, in late October, Congress passed a use-of-force authorization against Iraq,[95] a watershed moment in which our foreign policy focus officially shifted from

Afghanistan and avenging 9/11 to a muscular strategy of preemptive intervention.[96] Both of our New York senators at the time, Chuck Schumer and Hillary Clinton, voted for the authorization.[97] Their votes were a blow to those of us from the downtown community who felt that our safety and interests were not represented by those "yeas." The news reached me on a struggling computer as I dealt with a cigarette smoke crisis in my dorm and passed my days lobbying to switch rooms.

Starting school amid this war crisis required a delicate balancing act in my post-9/11 state, between hair-trigger anxiety that could flatten me for hours and my deep dismay at the implied and real violence being instigated by our national conversation. I wanted to express my frustration with the country's direction during the constant pseudo-intellectual rap sessions that peppered freshman orientation, but I had to be careful not to open the door to much discussion of foreign policy with unvetted new dorm mates and friends. I could handle disagreements intellectually, but I couldn't handle them emotionally. My passion for opposing war easily morphed into a directionless, helpless anger, a frustration that these new friends just didn't understand, and this often happened when I least expected it.

I was, at the same time, excited to share the activist part of my life with my new classmates. After a childhood spent attending labor and anti-war rallies with my mother, I was a pretty seasoned protester by the time my years at Vassar rolled around. As a child I had experienced demonstrations as almost always resulting in a lollipop or potentially a bouquet of colorful balloons, both favorable outcomes. By high school I would talk the ear off of anybody foolish enough to engage with me about the many times in history movements have won through collective action. I love protesting. I've always felt at home in a dense horde. I can read a crowd. I can lead a chant. I have informed opinions about policing tactics. I usually run into a friend or acquaintance somewhere along the route. I was, in short, an annoying person to attend your first march with.

Not realizing this, three new college friends agreed to join me at the first big anti-war rally of the Iraq War season on February 15, 2003. We traveled down to the city on Metro North, the commuter train line that ran between school and New York City. When major protests are planned, Metro North runs special unscheduled trains, dubbed "peace trains," so that the influx of protesters doesn't interrupt their usual service. We took photos on the train using our finicky digital cameras. I don't recognize myself in the photos—I'm bloated, acne peppers my face, the dark circles under my already deep-set eyes are, frustratingly, accentuated by the peace train's overhead fluorescent lighting. I'm dressed in a chaos of mismatched patterns and colors. I am, essentially, a poster child for how chronic stress manifests physically. My friends, by contrast, look young, healthy, and optimistic. They look like themselves.

On the ground at least, the protest felt like a meaningful turning point. For my friends, however, it was a rude introduction to the art of demonstrating. The rally was permitted in an unusual location, a narrow avenue on the East Side that wasn't near anything of importance. Michael Bloomberg had begun his first term as mayor the year before, but some familiar Giuliani-era crowd control tactics were still in full swing. Protesters split into small areas on either side of a wide emergency lane. By design, it was difficult to merge into the main body of the crowd; that meant that it was difficult to meet friends and difficult to leave the march if you needed to get out of the penned-off area that protesters were confined within. We hovered along the sides. Eventually, after a long effort and many dropped cell phone calls, we managed to meet up with a friend of mine from high school.

Because of the unusual setup, rallygoers spilled onto side streets and held mini-protests that weren't picked up in the official crowd estimates but felt as real as anything else. At one point, as our group of five searched for a way to get into the main protest area, we turned down a random block where hundreds of demonstrators were engaged in a bizarre face-off with a line of mounted police. The horses were bucking. The crowd was jeering. Tension hung in the air—it felt like the moment *just before* something dangerous happens. The crowd seemed like it was trapped there, but we were able to walk down the sidewalk and around the mounted police and nobody said a thing. We speedily exited to the safety of the empty intersection behind the standoff and stood there, unsure of where to go next.

Clever signs are part of what make a protest entertaining, but there were some unusually cynical ones propped up alongside the more common, repurposed sixties-era sign slogans, the ones that say things like "Bombing for Peace Is Like Fucking for Virginity." One less festive one that stuck with me read simply, "I Know Why They Hate Us." It was so spare and contemptuous, very unlike the plethora of quippy sayings that surrounded it. It was also impactful.

Our nation was, in that moment, acting like it wanted to be hated. We deployed rhetoric about supporting troops to send them into a dangerous and unnecessary conflict. We accused anti-war protesters, much like in the Vietnam era, of being unpatriotic while our president lied to us about the context of the war he was starting. We accused anybody who seemed even a little bit Muslim, code for being brown, of being a terrorist. Worst of all, some other kid's school was going to be stuck in the middle of a violent attack somewhere in the Middle East and we were going to justify it by invoking 9/11, by invoking my school.

My college friends saw what I was seeing, were exhilarated by the energy in the air and alarmed by the brooding, rageful tone of the crowd, but it wasn't personal for them in the same way it was for me. For them, at least from my vantage point, it was the exciting moment in which they stepped into the college experience they'd been promised. Many of their parents had, like mine, grown up in the Vietnam era and told stories of their own high school and college protesting days. My friends experienced that day as a chance to "be the change" for the first time.

For me, February 15 was an exorcism for my rage. I expended my nervous energy and anger from within a sea of New Yorkers who had shared some aspect of my experience. It was freezing cold and uncomfortable, but it was what I needed. I returned to Vassar exhausted but having reclaimed a little peace.

The next day's papers, carrying the official NYPD crowd estimates of one hundred thousand,[98] made it sound like not many people had attended, but that was not how it felt. The crowd was agitated and energetic and very, very angry, and there were a lot of us there—organizer estimates put the crowd at closer to 375,000,[99] and that doesn't account for the crowd that was just on the next block over, waiting to get in. Protests happened all over the world that day as well—at the time February 15 was heralded as the largest protest in history, with between 6 million and 11 million people participating in over 650 cities worldwide.[100]

AFTER MANY MONTHS OF hand-wringing about who had the power to declare war in the post–use-of-force era (Congress? The president? Divine intervention?), and who might support a war anyway if the wrong person made the call, President Bush officially declared war on Iraq on March 19, 2003.[101] On March 22 there was another rally.[102] I attended with my grandfather, a World War II veteran, social scientist, and notable slow walker who usually left the marching to us in favor of making scholarly declarations from home. He wore a sign that said, "Another veteran who thinks war is stupid," and moved at his snail's pace for half of the march before bowing out to recharge. He was a great source of encouragement when it came to radical thought, but that was the only time I ever actually protested with him. The crowds were a little overwhelming to a guy in his late eighties who'd broken his back while trying to touch his toes not too long ago, but he was very excited about it that evening. If we had been deeper into the social media age we would have probably appeared in a lot of photos. He'd be a meme by now.

IF A NATION AT war wasn't grounds for enough trauma, a new development on the domestic front occurred only a few months later, during the weeks I was preparing to move back into the dorms for my sophomore year at Vassar. It was a stressful time—my housing situation was in flux thanks to a very dramatic affair my roommate-to-be was having with an older man, my summer had been a wash professionally, and after an underwhelming first year, I wasn't all that eager to head back to school and try the whole "socializing while a mess" thing again. I had entered college eager to make the life-changing friendships people always talk about. Instead I was still speaking daily to my friends from Stuyvesant, still searching for those supposedly better college connections, the ones that were going to bring me to my tribe. My tribe was being awfully evasive.

In the midst of my back-to-school dread in August 2003, the EPA released an evaluation of its post-9/11 performance. In it, it conceded for the first time that when it "made the September 18 announcement that the air was 'safe' to breathe," it "did not have sufficient data and analyses to make the statement."[103] In essence, the press release was an admission that its leaders had lied to the people of Lower Manhattan. At the time I read it, I said, "No shit," and continued on with my packing, unfazed. I didn't realize that that little sentence would change everything about the dynamics of the 9/11 health discussion. There was immediate speculation about new lawsuits—several of them had already failed to make much of an impact, but this admission gave people new grounds to sue. There was also a developing interest in researching the downtown population, something community advocates had been fighting for for years.[104] About a month later, the World Trade Center Health Registry, a survey-based study intended to look into the health impacts of 9/11 on responders and the local community, began to recruit members of the downtown community.

I signed up for the registry in 2004 from my Vassar dorm room. The information must have come from my mother—she'd either seen it advertised on the subway or they'd sent a mailing to our house. Since more than half of the Stuyvesant classes that were there on 9/11 were away at college by the time they began collecting study participants, very few of my classmates found out about it in time to join. Of the tens of thousands of kids who were exposed to the WTC cleanup,[105] only about three thousand young adults exposed as children participated in the registry.[106]

The registry's initial survey was brutal. We were told it would be a thirty-minute telephone or in-person interview, and since I was at college, I elected to do it by phone. I didn't know anybody who had signed up, hadn't heard about anybody's survey experience, and didn't know what I was expecting the conversation to be. It just felt like an amorphous opportunity I couldn't overlook. A chance to make the case to *somebody* that what Stuyvesant students went through wasn't right. A chance to exorcise a little more of the anger I'd been sitting on. The program, however, didn't make that exorcism easy; it farmed out the interviews to a call service in the Deep South, and I remember not only straining to understand the operator as he asked me a slew of incredibly difficult questions but also thinking that he was talking outrageously slowly. I took the call alone from my sophomore-year dorm room, watching from the window as people played Frisbee out on the quad, pressing my early cell phone to my ear with a growing sense of unease, hoping it wouldn't run out of battery but also maybe that it would. Thanks to all the slow talking, the thirty-minute appointment took more than two hours, and I strained to understand questions like, "Are you having frequent disturbing memories of the events?" and, "Did you personally witness people jumping or falling?" They asked me what health effects I was experiencing and provided me with a litany of possible symptoms so that they might check something off of their list of the many possible health concerns. I hadn't yet thought about most of the conditions they listed, but I immediately began to. Constantly. The call with a stranger in the Deep South listing illnesses was a rude awakening to have at age twenty, as my dorm neighbors shouted down the halls, still feeling invincible and finding meaning in silly activities like guitar circles. Meanwhile, I was trapped in my dorm room with a monstrous burden.

Those early hiccups aside, the World Trade Center Health Registry currently stands as the largest post-disaster health registry in US history.[107] It's now mostly used to indicate potential areas of study for other researchers. As a self-reported study, it has limitations, but its establishment so early on was vital to our later efforts to get the health impacts of 9/11 taken seriously. It's one of the few sources of data on the people who lived, worked, or attended school downtown and is a primary reason that community members got included in later federal legislation geared toward first responders.

On that initial call, I was told that they expected as many as two hundred thousand people to enroll,[108] and while that was definitely an overstatement, the initial enrollment figures were still impressive—over seventy-one thousand people signed up.[109] Still, of the seventy-one thousand, only thirty-two hundred were children at the time of the attack.[110] Figuring out how to address and ameliorate the lack of young participants continues to be a discussion to this day, but having a start is better than not, even if that start was in a call center in the heavily accented Deep South.

THOUGH THE ANTI-WAR ORGANIZING continued, by 2004 attention had turned to the upcoming presidential race in which Senator John Kerry was running to unseat President George W. Bush. It was going to be my first chance to vote in a presidential election, and I'd be doing it from abroad—I was going to Athens, Greece, for the first semester of my junior year and Hanoi, Vietnam, for the second. Anything to get out of living at Vassar. Those life-changing college friendships had to be out there somewhere. Maybe they were in Europe or Asia.

Just before I left for Athens, I watched New York City briefly turn into a war zone again. Mayor Bloomberg had invited the Republican National Committee to host their presidential year convention at Madison Square Garden. It was hostile territory to say the least. By this point, given New Yorkers' widespread opposition to the GOP's foreign policy agenda in Iraq and the rest of the Middle East, the city had been turned via campaign messaging into more of a generic symbol than a place full of people who had directly suffered the losses of 9/11. Politically speaking, 9/11 stopped being about New Yorkers and started being about "New York," a place that might as well have had no people living in it. New Yorkers, meanwhile, were a menace in conservative rhetoric. The Twin Towers belonged to the nation; on the other hand, New Yorkers who didn't want to see the Twin Towers used to justify wars were unpatriotic. We did not belong to the nation in the same way.

Since I grew up close to Madison Square Garden, my entire neighborhood shut down during the RNC. For days my family participated in the protests—we marched, hosted people from out of town, provided a refuge and baked goods for tired protesters. When my parents weren't home, I'd find a collection of recovering activists lounging in our living room and assume my parents were still out there marching. Even my dad, who doesn't love crowds, helped the radical feminist anti-war group CODEPINK unfurl a huge banner from his office building and then helped them hide from the police so they wouldn't get arrested. I marched by with my mother in time to see the banner unfurl, excited to have an inside source.

The very decision to hold the RNC in New York City was among the most aggressive blows to post-9/11 New Yorkers in what was already a parade of insults. The scene felt dystopian. As GOP speakers aggressively invoked "New Yorkers" for our symbolic status inside Madison Square Garden, local protesters and unsuspecting bystanders were put under mass arrest just outside.[111]

Even among the frequent anti-war actions of the era, the 2004 RNC protests were notable for the high number of arrests—eighteen hundred in total.[112] The police used a new tactic in which they cornered groups of people, a tactic known as "kettling," then swept them up with plastic fencing and mass-detained them. Police then transported detainees to a holding facility in a bus station on an isolated pier where they'd spend hours, sometimes days, awaiting processing.[113] An NYPD surveillance operation that began targeting anti-war activists as early as 2003 led to some of the detained being hit with trumped-up charges.[114] Onlookers and tourists were accidentally swept up with startling frequency. Years later, in 2014, the city wound up paying an astounding $17.9 million settlement to the protesters whose civil rights they had violated.[115]

When the local news started covering the mass arrests, the GOP was ultimately put on blast—not because the convention was an insult to New Yorkers, though. In sweeping up shoppers and bystanders, the GOP was committing a cardinal New York sin: being bad for business. You don't mess with money in New York.

AFTER A WEEK OF marching I left for Greece, where I continued to attend anti-war marches. A few months later I voted in my first presidential election from the cozy common room of my study abroad program in Athens. I did, as it turned out, find some tribe members there. Some surprising ones, even. I cast my first presidential ballot while sitting beside a conservative friend, Rebecca. We supported different candidates—she voted for President George W. Bush and I voted for Senator John Kerry—but we both loved debating and loved voting, so we were happy for each other anyway.

Though a few of my male friends had tried to launch political rebellions against their liberal parents in our mid-teens, Rebecca was the first true believer I was ever close to—a legacy Republican and proud. We had a lot of interesting conversations that year thanks to that election. Both of us came from schools at which the student body had pretty consistent political views—she attended a Catholic university at which opposition to abortion was pro forma, while Vassar was known for its hippy nonsense and leftward leanings. We breached our political divide because Rebecca was, aside from being funny and intelligent, generous and open to discussing our political differences. I tried to be the same. A few months after we made those presidential votes, in true idealist-college-student form, I sat her down at a café and said, "Just hear me out. I think you may be a socialist." She didn't grant me that, but she did leave the program that semester a different person politically. She started the Democrats club at her school the next year.

I also left that semester a different person politically. My friendship with Rebecca helped me hone in on an incredibly valuable skill, one that I'd need in my later political endeavors. I learned from her how to talk about politics with people I don't agree with. When people in the intervening years have told me I should run for office (it happens a lot), I'm pretty sure it's not because they think I'd be great at dealing with nasty negotiations. I'd be awful at it. What I'm good at is communicating what's at stake on a given issue to people who hold different views and priorities. Talking to Rebecca, I learned how to find commonalities, even when pointing out differences. I now regularly talk about politics in rideshares, on airplanes, in bus stations. I never worry that I'll make it awkward, and it rarely is (my Lyft passenger score is perfect!), but this confidence took practice. The skill that is handling disagreement gracefully evaded me for a bit after 9/11, but by 2004 I had started to find it again, and that semester talking politics with Rebecca was critical. It was, in many ways, also central to why, in 2006, I decided that I should talk about 9/11 and health care. Tethering myself to a challenging issue, an issue that brings up terrible memories for both me and my classmates, was something that I was willing and, most importantly, able to do while others were not. I found the widespread gaslighting and denialism around 9/11 health issues as frustrating as everybody else, but my secret power was my willingness to patiently hang on until I found the opening where I could tell somebody that they should believe me and, maybe also, that they might be a socialist.

There were other reasons behind my willingness to get involved in the 9/11 health discussions too. One was that Dr. Ting, right after 9/11, confirmed that he didn't think the air was safe, so I'd had that fact in my back pocket even when school officials told us the opposite and students, desperate to believe it, started to repeat that false fact. Having confirmation of a truth from a credible source, even if it's just a faint memory from a conversation years ago, is helpful when you're being gaslit. It propelled me to look for evidence, which was being quietly accumulated by other members of the community, that proved my suspicions. I'd also made it into the health registry, which few of my classmates had accomplished because they weren't in town to see the advertisements and receive the notices before the study closed to new participants. I was asthmatic before 9/11, so I had plenty of familiarity with how seemingly minor air pollution can impact a person's respiratory health in dramatic ways. I knew that if a house cat could send me to the emergency room—where inevitably a doctor would show me an X-ray of my lungs and the scar tissue that comes with just being a run-of-the-mill asthmatic—then surely a massive environmental disaster would have an impact on my long-term health.

Being asthmatic also gave me another admittedly depressing advantage—an in-depth understanding of how the health care laws in America work and, often, don't work. I've always had a preexisting condition, that nasty American insurance industry term that marks you as a vulnerable and undesirable customer.[116] Before insurance discrimination against people with preexisting conditions was outlawed in 2010 by the Affordable Care Act (ACA), insurance companies would do whatever they could to avoid insuring people who might require costly care.[117] Just a few years after I graduated from college, amid a major national discussion about health care reform, the House Oversight Committee found that the top-four for-profit insurers were denying coverage to, on average, one in seven applicants on the basis of preexisting conditions, though for some companies, the ratio was as low as one in three.[118] Conditions as common as diabetes and heart disease would often trigger automatic denials, as would health situations as central to the human experience as pregnancy.[119] It was legal for insurers to deny coverage to domestic violence and rape victims on the basis that their victimization was a preexisting conditions.[120] Just before the health care reforms of 2010, a four-month-old baby was denied insurance for being "too fat."[121] The system was preposterous.

By 2006, while many college students had continued along merrily, health concern–free and therefore unaware of this lurking danger, I'd already put in years of worrying about my future health care costs thanks to my asthma. The year I graduated from college predated the Affordable Care Act, which, beyond protecting those with preexisting conditions, allowed children to stay on their parents' health plans until the age of twenty-six.[122] In 2006, the year I graduated, college students left school without health insurance and no state had yet figured out a good solution to protect consumers from discrimination in the individual health care marketplace. In New York, a company couldn't spike your premiums or refuse you coverage unless you'd had a gap in coverage of longer than sixty-two days,[123] but as a result, insurance premiums regularly topped $500 a month for even young healthy people.[124] (If you did have a gap in coverage, companies could refuse to cover your preexisting conditions, meaning you'd pay $500 a month and not even get coverage for the one concern you knew you'd need care for.) In California, premiums were lower, but insurance companies could reject you outright simply for having a preexisting condition.[125] There, being sick with anything in the individual insurance market meant you might not be able to get insurance at all.

I began stockpiling my asthma medicine, which cost over $300 a month, at the beginning of my senior year of college. I would take it half as often as prescribed, then lie to my doctor about it. I kept my extra Advair canisters at the back of my closet, hidden, as if they were my most precious possession. Periodically I opened my closet just to count them and, by extension, the number of months of breathing I had left. By the end of my senior year I had about a six-month supply that I could make last almost a year if I cut down my dosing further and continued to receive the occasional sample from a doctor, using the medicine as intended only during bad allergy seasons or weeks where cats were in my life. I operated against medical advice because it was the only way I could keep using the drug that kept me healthy. It left me vulnerable to colds and allergies, which could knock me off my feet for weeks or even months, but it was better than being at risk of running out.

A FEW MONTHS BEFORE graduation, I attended a seminar for seniors put on by Vassar's Career Development Office. The topic was benefits, which meant they had to entice the audience with free food. I was one of the few people who attended eagerly. Since most of us would be booted off of our parents' health insurance the moment we were handed a diploma, the school's presentation was meant to give us a sense of what we should do next. It began with an upbeat listing of the types of jobs we might get after graduation. It was 2006, two years before the massive economic collapse of 2008 and the failures of several large banks, so the school was particularly intrigued by the wealth of opportunities available in investment banking.

We were assured that, should we pursue work in the glamorous, high-paying financial sector, the benefits package would be great and we'd have nothing to worry about. The small print, which they rushed by, was that this would be the case only if we started work right away. There was also the unspoken trade-off we'd be making, which we whispered about based on the tales of recent graduates. Investment banking might give us insurance, but it would also require 120-hour workweeks spent staring at spreadsheets; the high-dollar bonuses would be paid alongside the "opportunity" to engage in fun office antics like sneaking your coat out in a FedEx box to avoid looking like you were leaving for the day as bleary-eyed analysts competed with you to seem like the most productive and dedicated staffers. Most of my classmates who did take those jobs would lose them within a couple of years and be back on the benefits market, but alas.

If it seemed odd for the administration at a liberal arts school famous for its art history department to be hard-selling jobs in finance to its relatively unstructured and vegan-forward student body, it became clear why they'd done it in the second half of the presentation. That half was about what to do if you either didn't get a job (the non-finance economy was already starting to buckle) or were planning to intern (i.e., work for no pay), freelance (planning to freelance was often what people like me who didn't like spreadsheets said they were doing, but it wasn't much of a plan), or get one of those humanities jobs that don't offer any benefits or really much in the way of pay. Their answer was simple: panic.

As the seminar wore on and the cookies ran out, it became clear that the school didn't have much helpful advice for the bulk of us who would not cut it at Morgan Stanley. They most certainly couldn't help anybody who might face discrimination on the insurance market because they were already sick. Their point of view seemed to be that since we'd played the game well enough to get into a good college, we might as well stick to the rules and get into the even more competitive good jobs market. People who couldn't hack it didn't deserve Advair.

I walked out terrified. I'd never really taken to life at Vassar—it was too insular, more like the prep schools I'd read about in novels than the collegiate experience I'd expected. Suddenly, however, I became very nervous about leaving.

TO ADD TO MY many fears about life outside the ivory tower: just around the time that I attended the benefits seminar, I learned about the death of James Zadroga. Back in the spring of 2006, an emerging health crisis among 9/11 first responders started to get some play in the media, and Zadroga, an NYPD officer and 9/11 responder who died in January 2006 from lung disease,[126] was at the center of the controversy. Questions swirled about his cause of death and whether it might be related to his service at Ground Zero. Because of this speculation, the downtown air quality conversation, which until that point had been taking place primarily among a cadre of activists working in New York City, began to bubble up in media coverage elsewhere. Those of us outside the city were able to take notice of it for the first time. This was just a month before a group of residents and office workers announced that they were suing the Environmental Protection Agency for misleading people by telling them that the air in Lower Manhattan was safe to breathe.[127]

In April 2006, a pathologist at the medical examiner's office in Ocean County, New Jersey, made an astonishing assertion that supported the speculation—James Zadroga's cause of death, lung disease at age thirty-four, was ruled to be directly related to his exposures as a first responder on 9/11.[128] This made him the very first responder to have his death directly linked to the air at Ground Zero. By August of that year, in response to massive local pressure, then New York governor George Pataki signed into law some early protections for first responders.[129]

Though few people were discussing the Lower Manhattan community's World Trade Center exposures outside of Lower Manhattan itself, the connection between Zadroga's experience and mine was not lost on me as I tried to strategize my way through the postcollege benefits apocalypse. If toxic air at the cleanup site had caused a thirty-four-year-old policeman to die, why should kids who went to school there in that same period be struggling to figure out if they'd even be able to see a doctor in the first place? The thought bounced around in my head for days as I grew angrier and angrier at its implication.

There were, by the way, attempts to debunk Zadroga's cause-of-death declaration in the ensuing years. The city, under Mayor Michael Bloomberg, did not want to admit that the air in Lower Manhattan was toxic when one hundred thousand responders were sent there to work, perhaps because so many of those responders were city employees.[130] The next year the New

York City medical examiner's office tried to walk back the Ocean County office's claims and assert that Zadroga's cause of death was self-injection of ground-up prescription drugs, attempting to paint him as a drug abuser.[131] A third opinion, which Zadroga's family sought from New York State Police chief forensic pathologist Dr. Michael Baden, supported the initial declaration that the cause of death was 9/11 since,[132] as the *New York Daily News* put it, "Zadroga had a type of 'black lung' disease typically seen in coal miners and caused by inhaling particulate matter. Under a microscope, 'You could see glass fibers there,' Baden said. 'You don't get that from injecting drugs.'"[133] Touché.

FOR MY PART, I struggled a lot with what to do with a growing, silent alarm that left me in a state of persistent crisis—chronically indecisive about how to approach a future that felt more like an ominous threat than a promising opportunity. A future in which I saw myself spending all my time working just to afford the mounting costs of a growing list of 9/11-related health needs. Who cares about careers when you're looking at that kind of perma-misery? I wanted to take action to stave off the fear.

Unsure of where to start, I looked to my primary role model for all things action-related, my mother. A decade prior she had scored a major victory and gotten an op-ed published in *The New York Times* during a labor dispute between the city and her union, the United Federation of Teachers.[134] Inspired by her success, I began a bizarre ritual of writing op-eds from my dorm room whenever I was politically frustrated. Naturally, they never got published since they were mostly the political rantings of a PTSD-stricken twenty-year-old, but the Zadroga and community health situation seemed a worthy topic for another op-ed, so I began to plan an essay. As I procrastinated on finishing it, though, I had a kind of wacky idea. I decided to try a new tact.

One evening, in a blaze of rageful glory, I sat down and wrote a letter about the situation to a theoretical list of public officials, names TBD. I sent it to a small group of friends from Stuyvesant to gauge their response, assuming that they wouldn't have much of a reaction but knowing that the exercise of sending it *somewhere* was central to my ability to feel good about the effort. Having a readership would, on some level, make the act of writing feel active instead of passive and unproductive. It would make the whole thing more than just a self-help exercise. I decided to aim high with what I was asking for, demanding health care for the kids of Ground Zero for the rest of our lives, full stop. The very first response I got was from a good friend, now a lawyer at a fancy white-shoe firm in DC, whose enthusiastic endorsement of the letter was a little surprising to me. I thought he'd be in favor of a more measured approach, a smaller ask, a less abrasive tone. He was a small-government guy in those days, one of the people toying with the idea of rebelling against his family by becoming a Republican. When he said he was in, that he'd be willing to add his name to the letter, I realized I had hit on something. More responses followed, most saying they'd be happy to add their names too. I sent the email to a few more people and got the same positive replies. Then, I started thinking bigger.

Facebook was relatively new on the scene in 2006, having launched just two years earlier as TheFacebook.com;[135] it was a trendier version of the social media predecessors we were using back then. Unlike Myspace and Friendster (aw, Friendster), Facebook was appealing because it was a college-only service that was expanding school by school—it wasn't yet open to parents or younger siblings. The college-only focus made it an ideal way to contact former Stuyvesant alumni, most of whom were attending four-year colleges that were already served by the platform. Facebook didn't offer much beyond the very bare-bones profiles standard of its forebears, but it allowed me to search by high school and class year and find many of my former Stuyvesant classmates.

I posted the letter on the free blogging platform Blogger on March 31, 2006,[136] and began messaging Stuyvesant alumni between classes and paper-writing, hitting them twenty to thirty at a time, asking them to add their names by either replying to my message or commenting on the post. I titled the post "Open Letter," and added an exclamation-point-heavy note at the top for alumni so they could share it with friends. The petition letter started to get some traffic.

To Whom It May Concern,

On February 2 a federal judge found the former head of the Environmental Protection Agency Christie Whitman culpable enough to stand trial for putting the public in danger by making misleading statements about the air quality in Lower Manhattan after the attacks of September 11, thus upholding a class action suit filed on behalf of residents and schoolchildren in downtown Manhattan and Brooklyn. Students at Stuyvesant High School were among the many that were directly affected by the misinformation released by the Environmental Protection Agency under her leadership. We had the additional misfortune of being the first students called back to Lower Manhattan after the attacks. At the time, fires were still burning at the World Trade Center site and debris was being taken to the landfill by way of a barge located directly outside our school building. We had several fire drills in our first days back that informed us of our new emergency route, which led us even closer to the burning debris at the site of the destruction (our old emergency route up West St. was being blocked by the barge and a large crane). Although the Board of Education continually assured us of the safety of the air at our school, the smell of smoke was strong every afternoon for months after the attacks. Parents were told at the first PTA meeting after our return, that nobody, even those of us with respiratory health concerns, would be able to leave Stuyvesant for the duration of the cleanup process; we had to stay or would forfeit our spots at the school. Given the effort most of us put into getting into Stuyvesant, leaving was not an option.

Eventually, we learned that the school building had not been cleaned as thoroughly as promised.

Most of the Stuyvesant students that were seniors in the year of the attacks are graduating from college this year. We are entering a world in which jobs are scarce, starting pay is low, and public benefits are dwindling. As you know, health coverage is expensive and difficult to obtain, especially on a starting salary. More Americans go bankrupt as a result of health expenses than over any other issue, and the current Administration is making very little effort to make obtaining health coverage any easier or more affordable. Additionally, as college students and soon-to-be graduates, many of us have already accrued large amounts of debt to pay for our educations.

As the canaries used to promote the revitalization of downtown Manhattan after 9/11, we were given no choice but to accept the health risks that went along with attending school in Lower Manhattan in the 2001/2002 school year. Ms. Whitman's assurances were a very relevant part of why we were permitted to return to our building, which had been used as the command center for the rescue effort at Ground Zero, only a month after September 11, on October 9, 2001. Our administrators and teachers already have health coverage. As students, we don't. As victims of 9/11, and, especially, victims of Ms. Whitman's misinformation campaign, we served as "draftees" in the media campaign to reassure the American people. At the least, in recognition of the risks we undertook simply by attending school, we should be guaranteed health insurance for the rest of our lives. It is imperative that you support us in this effort. We request your help in meeting this goal, ideally by supporting the introduction of legislation toward this end.

Sincerely,
Lila Nordstrom[137]

THE LETTER RACKED UP an additional 150 names pretty quickly and incited only a few angry comments from people who thought I should stop taking the attention away from first responders. I sent the letter on April 3, 2006, to local officials, members of the New York congressional delegation, and a DC lawyer named Richard Ben-Veniste, though I continued to add names to the petition as they came, already planning for a second mailing.

The first response was from Ben-Veniste, a Stuyvesant alumnus who, before 9/11, was most famous for his role as chief of the Watergate Task Force.[138] He'd been retained by the Stuyvesant Parents' Association during their early 2002 attempt to sue the city over the school's environmental conditions,[139] and in 2003 he was tapped to be a member of the 9/11 Commission, a bipartisan ten-person committee set up by the federal government in November 2002 to provide a complete account of how the attacks of 9/11 had happened and what we could do to be better prepared in the future.[140] Ben-Veniste was known for asking tough questions of the administration, which is why I chose to contact him. He commended me for bringing attention to the issue and told me he was keeping an eye on the court cases going forward. Already the petition was getting more of a response than my op-ed writing.

After some follow-up, I was also able to set up a call with Representative Jerrold Nadler's chief of staff, Amy Rutkin. She wasn't incredibly optimistic about the chance that federal legislation would pass under the Bush administration but filled me in on the details. Representative Nadler, whom I had met a few times with my mother in the course of her own community work, was passing through as she made the call and asked a few questions on the line. Stuyvesant and Ground Zero were in Nadler's district, and he is a Stuyvesant alumnus as well. Because of this, he was better versed than many of his colleagues on the particulars of the Stuyvesant experience and the air quality concerns at the school during the WTC cleanup. They promised they'd keep me updated but didn't see much chance that our demand for health coverage would be met—at least not in the near future.

One thing that I have learned to appreciate over the years about Nadler's office and Amy Rutkin in particular is that, while they are very good at the constituent services side of their job, they're always direct and honest about the political realities they, and by extension their constituents, are facing. It's helpful to know these realities when you're heading into political battle.

AT THE END OF April, just before I graduated from Vassar, the United for Peace and Justice coalition held yet another big anti-war march, and my mother got word that her favorite marching companions, the Raging Grannies, would be coming into the city for it. The Raging Grannies is a group with several chapters around New York State in which women of all ages dress up as caricaturesque grannie figures (with quilted aprons, doilies, etc.) and sing familiar songs rewritten as anti-war anthems.[141] They were a big hit on the early 2000s anti-war circuit, attracting lots of crowd attention as they strolled down the street pushing a cart with a speaker and handing out lyric sheets. My mother, who loves to sing and jumps at any political theater opportunity, marched with them at the RNC protests in 2004 and had joined them at various protests since. She would only march with them when the Rochester Raging Grannies were in town—she claimed the New York City Raging Grannies weren't as much fun—so our house was often turned into a staging area where out-of-town grannies could get into costume. My mother dressed in quilting scraps and oversize aprons (she's 4'10", so all aprons are oversize on her) for their performances, often carrying the tune for the others with her loud and proud singing.

At the April 29 march, the grannies were given a rare opportunity— they were invited to perform during the kickoff speeches and to walk at the very front of the peace march.[142] That meant the grannies were allowed into the cordoned-off area housing the "lead contingent," the movement's noncontroversial term for the VIP section. My mother snuck me in with her so that I could hit up some of the politicians I'd mailed the letter to.

As a Nordstrom, I'd been trained well for this kind of guerilla lobbying—my mother never shied away from inundating politicians with her thoughts regardless of whether we were in their office or on a random street corner. Inside the lead contingent area I made my way around the crowd, shaking hands and introducing myself to anybody I recognized. If appropriate, I'd tell them that I had just sent their office a petition related to 9/11. I talked to a lot of people that day whom I never thought I'd meet. Famed civil rights attorney Norman Siegel, the former executive director of the New York Civil Liberties Union and frequent Giuliani courtroom opponent,[143] was there, so I spoke to him and took his card so we could set up a meeting. I also approached Manhattan borough president Scott Stringer. Our conversation turned out to be the big prize.

Scott Stringer had initially struck people as a very random addition to my list of recipients, but I included him for a reason—he was ubiquitous. If I happened to be at an event for any of the city's Democratic clubs (my parents were on-again, off-again members of several clubs over the course of my lifetime), he'd be there. If I happened to check out a local news story, he'd be quoted. He was a nice guy, still connected to the neighborhood in a meaningful way, but his mandate as Manhattan borough president was vague so he had time for me in a way that, say, Speaker of the City Council Christine Quinn (my own city council representative) did not.

A former state assemblyman from the Upper West Side, Stringer was widely considered to be a protégé of Congressman Nadler. The two of them used to campaign together outside of the original Fairway Market on the Upper West Side, and I'd met him there more than once. My mom usually introduced me as if they were old friends, though I'm not positive Stringer knew her as anything other than one of the many little loud ladies in the area to avoid. He was always gracious enough to play along nonetheless, and those Fairway meetings were formative for me in a lot of ways. It was outside Fairway that I first learned to treat politicians as my equal, not as celebrities deigning to shake my hand. My mother introduced "Scott" and

"Jerry" by their first names. This made them seem significantly less intimidating when I started to approach them on my own. When I stuck my hand out to Scott Stringer at that April 29 protest, I didn't get swept up in honorifics. I opened with, "Scott, I'm Lila Nordstrom. We've met." Worked like a charm.

The borough presidents in New York are holdovers from another era. The job has been largely robbed of its teeth—borough presidents can propose legislation to the city council but they can't vote on it—so a lot of what they do is raise the profiles of local issues that are being overlooked. It's a useful role, because borough presidents can dig into issues that go beyond specific policy fixes and coordinate with city and state agencies even when there isn't going to be a legislative victory to announce. Basically, Stringer was a guy who could raise the profile of my issue with not just his constituents but also the other people on the letter's recipient list and the media. When I introduced myself, he took an immediate interest. He heard my concerns and promised me a meeting right away. In a rare turn of events, he actually delivered. We quickly set up a meeting for the following Friday.

After the protest and before the meeting I sent an update to the petition signees, hoping to seize on the momentum of the moment. In it I encouraged them to pass the petition letter along and updated them about my political successes, but I also added a new request—that people get involved beyond just signing. After recounting the results of my guerilla advocacy, I asked the list for volunteers to join me for a potential meeting with Norman Siegel.

Then, of course, there were the legislative updates, and a clumsy attempt to be transparent about what Nadler's office had told me about Stuyvesant's media appeal:

> I also spoke to the Chief of Staff at Rep. Nadler's New York
> office. Amy Rutkin, who I talked to, had a long conversation with
> me about our case. Their legislative aides are looking into ways

to introduce health legislation but are having a hard time even with emergency worker cases. She did say, however, that the Stuyvesant case would play very well in the news and therefore that they could probably get us some publicity which would increase the chance that their office could then introduce legislation, etc. Also, in the event that legislation getting us health insurance isn't possible in this particular Congress (it's Republican controlled, Nadler's a Democrat, enough said), she did mention the idea of setting up some kind of monitoring program for us to find out if we do get health problems due to 9/11. Nadler was sitting next to her during the phone call and asked me questions through her during the call so he'll remember the conversation and knows about our case.

If anybody has any other political contacts, please let me know or contact them yourself with information. Also, anybody that wants to be more involved in general, even if you don't want to meet with Norman Siegel, etc., please let me know.

MY MEETING WITH SCOTT STRINGER was not the first occasion for which I'd been into the Municipal Building, a goliath across the street from City Hall that overlooks the Brooklyn Bridge, but it was my first visit since the age of five, when I attended my parents' wedding there, waiting for our turn in a dingy room full of pregnant ladies in elaborate white dresses. Stringer's office was on the nineteenth floor, and the views were fantastic.

Stringer and his chief of staff sat with me in Stringer's comically large and rather furniture-light office and listened to me talk about the Stuyvesant experience after 9/11. I began with the usual.

"We were only out of school for a few weeks. We came back downtown on October 9, which wasn't even a month after the attacks."

It took a moment for him to work out what that meant. To remember what the neighborhood had looked like and smelled like back in October

2001, five years prior, before he was even charged with representing it. Finally, he asked, "It was that soon?"

I laid on new facts from there, telling him that they didn't clear the air ducts until the following summer. And we were right next to the debris barge. And they weren't even hosing down the debris. It was just being dumped right next to our air intake system all day. A literal toxic waste dump next to a school.

He expressed surprise and asked why it was allowed.

I didn't have a good answer for him. "In the name of returning to normalcy, I guess?" was all I could think to say. The real answer was plain negligence, but I wasn't sure how city officials would react to that word. I didn't want him to feel implicated, even as somebody who wasn't representing the area at the time, in a way that made him unwilling to help us.

He asked me why nobody was talking about this.

I shrugged. "We went to war and forgot about this stuff."

Stringer's primary shock rooted in the fact that this was all new information to him, but he wasn't in the dark alone. In the chaos of the last four years, it felt like very few people had grappled with how many lives were unexpectedly impacted by the World Trade Center cleanup. When we were swept into war, first responders became the face of the 9/11 conversation. It was easy to make connections between first responders and soldiers. In a public discourse that was still embroiled in a nasty "you're either with us or against us" rhetoric, it was patriotic to care about them. Community concerns failed to get much of an airing after that, and the scale of the community concerns was much broader and deeper than anybody would have guessed. Asking people to reframe their understanding of the 9/11 cleanup so that it included people as unlike first responders as children was a weighty request.

Stringer's staff got to work immediately. They announced that they were seeking public and private funds to get us included in a small 9/11 screening program for uninsured community members at Bellevue

Hospital.[144] Mayor Bloomberg, around that time, announced that the city would allocate $16 million to expand the program over the next five years as well.[145] Stringer's staff then put me in touch with some of the other activists working on this issue and helped me get in contact with the city, state, and federal officials I'd sent the letter to, as well as others who happened to be Stuyvesant alumni.

Thanks to their interventions, I soon had updates from another one of the New York City congressional offices leading on the issue, that of Congresswoman Carolyn Maloney. Her staff told me they had legislation sitting in committee, but the bill had been stagnant since 2004 so nobody was feeling that optimistic. Buried in that call was a tidbit of information that I didn't expect, however. I learned that there were, bizarrely, two competing bills tackling the 9/11 health issue—Nadler and Maloney had proposed different solutions to treating the affected community. That was a layer of complication that felt almost Kafkaesque. A puzzle within a puzzle. As if passing a unified bill wouldn't be hard enough. I wasn't yet interested in wading into the discord.

Just after the Stringer meeting, I attended my college graduation. I don't really remember who Vassar's speaker was that year, maybe because those of us who get to have a Bill Clinton at our high school graduations become spoiled and insufferable, but also because the entire process was a blur. I was eager to leave Poughkeepsie and ready to move on with my life. I was also nervously undecided about what kind of life I wanted to have. The petition gave me a kind of calling, which was helpful because the vast expanse of adulthood staring me in the face did not seem to be providing easy answers. My short-term plan was to kill time until I figured out whether I had a long-term plan.

In May I moved back to New York City and in with my parents, reasoning that I'd rather live in the center of Manhattan rent-free than pay more money than I had ever seen in my life to live forty-five minutes deep into one of the outer boroughs. I worked part-time at a small nonprofit and part-time at a fake job in my dad's office that mostly involved snacking and perusing the internet for no pay and a fake title on my résumé. I pondered moving to California, where my closest friend was beginning a writing career, but wasn't sure I had the guts, so I bided my time and stayed put and, in the meantime, did what I had been trained to do since birth. I rabble-roused.

As my Stuyvesant friends all diligently went out and got real jobs and made sometimes misguided attempts at starting their lives, I passed time following up on the petition, strategizing about how to get media attention, and collecting signatures. Then, that fall, some horrible news broke the whole case wide open. One of my classmates had just been diagnosed with cancer, and he believed it to be 9/11-related.

CHAPTER 7

ANOTHER SEPTEMBER

The first cancer report felt like a bomb dropping. There is no satisfaction in being right about young people getting cancer. No joy in the "I told you so."

The news arrived in September in an innocent email, a response to a query. In some ways it felt small and unverified, difficult to extrapolate anything from. What does one cancer mean? Can't anybody get cancer? Genes are a crapshoot. Pollution is everywhere. People are unlucky sometimes.

In the meetings I'd taken so far, I'd been talking about the threat of cancer, but subconsciously I'd been hoping my rhetoric was hyperbolic. Hoping when I told people I was worried about the future, that our exposures were not really that bad, that I was just a dramatic kid overreacting. Hoping that we'd just get asthma, maybe suffer chronic coughs, and be done with it. Cancer is not some average, everyday chronic but manageable illness. It's unpredictable. It's deadly. We talk about recovery from cancer using fighting metaphors. Nobody has ever asked me to "beat" asthma. Many doctors have, instead, talked to me about how to live *with* it. You can't live *with* cancer. You can only get rid of it or die from it.

Back when I was only talking about theoretical cancers, I tried to project an upbeat, active demeanor in interviews and meetings about 9/11. I wanted to use my youth and relatively good health to show I had the energy to keep fighting. My platform was mostly theoretical. It was about justice for the kids of 9/11, not justice for the current victims of fatal disease. A real cancer is an inherently more serious thing.

Even before the cancer story blew up, by the middle of 2006, some media interest in my efforts was already starting to percolate. That summer, deep into my career as an office-sitter-slash-reader-of-blogs, I was contacted by a reporter from *The Village Voice*, Kristen Lombardi. She was covering a slew of 9/11 health stories, and somebody had forwarded her my petition. I read her email in between Apartment Therapy posts, not really comprehending how big a break her interest could be for us. I replied casually that I'd be happy to talk.

Conversations about the nonresponders living, working, and attending school in Lower Manhattan after 9/11 had hit local media in fits and starts. Most of the focus was on the people living in the area immediately surrounding the WTC site, an upper-middle-class, well-organized community with heavy exposures and a helpful smattering of angry, white middle-class parents. The national discussion was fully responder-focused when it existed at all, but local politicians would periodically throw a haphazard press conference or event and talk about the people who lived downtown. It was, after all, where their constituents were. It was where their votes came from.

I didn't always retain the details of what was going on in the community, but a few things had broken through the noise. At a press conference in mid-July, Lower Manhattan city councilmember Alan Gerson asked for $5 million in seed money to launch a clinic for Lower Manhattan residents suffering from 9/11-related conditions.[146] Gerson, like Nadler a Stuyvesant alum from a previous era, was hoping to encourage the Lower Manhattan Development Corporation (LMDC), the city-state agency in charge of redeveloping the WTC site, to fund the clinic.[147] The unspoken charge, the reason this effort was politically expedient, was that LMDC had been directly responsible for many resident exposures.[148] They had offered financial incentives to people to encourage them to move into Battery Park City, just to the west of Ground Zero, before the WTC cleanup was fully over.[149] These tax breaks, grants, and rent incentives, equal to 30 percent off of monthly rent for those moving into the areas most affected by the disaster,[150] were some of the many post-9/11 choices that placed the nation's perceived economic needs—the need to get things back to normal—over those of the people actually living and working downtown.

Conversation about the clinic bounced around in the local news for a while, but the conception of who composed the community seemed pretty narrow, limited mostly to residents of Battery Park City and environs. When children were mentioned, it was usually by parents of young kids who lived in the neighborhood. When adults were quoted, they were from Community Board 1, the political body that represented the district's residents. The thousands of students who were commuting in and out of the area were generally not mentioned or consulted.

When I finally spoke to Lombardi, she said she was eager to find a new angle on the 9/11 health story. I pitched her a story about the nonresident student experience after 9/11 and offered to put her in touch with some classmates who had signed the petition.

We had a new name for our project by this point, StuyHealth, which was agreed upon by the list of signees after an early July email update. It wasn't necessarily clever, but it was an improvement over my unwieldy previous iteration, the Stuyvesant Healthcare Initiative. Starting a project like StuyHealth without a plan is a good way to learn what your strengths and weaknesses are. I was, as it turned out, good at messaging, good at being a pest to political staffers, and bad at branding. Lesson learned.

Lombardi seemed interested, but her first question was a query I still dread from reporters. It's also the first thing I'm asked in every interview.

"How many of you are sick?"

The question seeks an obvious first point of reference, but in the survivor community and at Stuyvesant in particular, our relationship to the illness data is a little complicated. To put it bluntly, nobody was monitoring our health then, just as nobody is monitoring our health now.

There are a couple of incomplete programs that get data on survivors, including the World Trade Center Health Registry and the World Trade Center Health Program, a federal treatment program established several years after Lombardi and I spoke,[151] but neither offers this kind of holistic data. They both have very limited cohorts, cohorts that are especially lacking in young adults. The honest answer to her question, both in 2006 and years later, is, "I don't know."

Why I don't know goes deeper than just what conditions and people are and are not being monitored for, too. There is also not, nor has there ever been, a definitive list of linked conditions. There is simply a growing list that morphs and changes as research continues. Monitoring only works if you're looking for the right clues.

For the most part, finding out who was sick back then and who is sick now is a project conducted via word of mouth, just as the project of finding out what people are sick with is an inexact science. Around the time of the initial petition, I started getting random emails from former classmates alerting me to unusual health issues they'd faced. A lot of the issues seemed like they could be related, but by that point we didn't have proof that anything was, just that we were wary and right to be scared. By the end of 2007, my standard reply was, "I'll add this to the list." Within a few years the list included a number of reproductive health issues ranging from uterine cysts to unexplained miscarriages, autoimmune issues like scleroderma, chronic pain, spontaneous anaphylaxis, a litany of bizarre respiratory and gastrointestinal concerns, and, of course, cancers, which were mostly leukemias and lymphomas by that point. Some of the conditions that affected large numbers of my classmates have still never been definitively linked by research to the attacks, though I've gathered in conversation with other advocates and doctors that they will likely be linked in the future.

I didn't have most of this information when I got the call from Lombardi. We were lucky that she was a serious investigative journalist and seemed interested in doing a longer series of stories about the issue, not just a quick sensationalistic news piece. Her first article was going to focus on our exposures and my organizing efforts. It would be a major feature in the print edition of *The Village Voice*. We spoke at length, gathering information and sources for weeks. Talking to Lombardi was my first attempt at pitching the petition, the Stuyvesant experience, and the experience of students in general—those of us who didn't really need to be down there—directly to press. It was exciting and validating. It gave me a reason to contact classmates and announce that the StuyHealth project was going well. That they could trust me to carry the weight of this topic in a way that was inclusive and responsible and gave them all a chance to weigh in.

I was new to the movement PR game, though. The interviews and updates continued on a positive note for a while, but as our correspondence bled into the following days, then weeks, then months, the holdup began to concern me. Sensing that something was amiss, I started to ask the questions that I had the creeping sense I didn't really want the answers to, like when was the story going to print? I avoided even raising the subject for weeks. Lombardi continued to assure me it was happening; she was just called out to work on something else. She was pulled into a new topic. She had to travel. Then, of course, her editor nixed the story. He said it was because young adults weren't sick enough. The implication: Our story just wasn't exciting enough to compete with responder illness narratives. *Sorry.*

Years later, in a completely unrelated but parallel life, I spent three years working at a major talent agency in Los Angeles. Up until that point, I'd spent years trying to get a writing agent and failing, watching people around me who were both more and less talented get signed. I listened diligently to the advice of people who'd found success and reflected back to me a system that was, despite its many flaws, relatively meritocratic. Not in every way, not in every case, but no matter how much reality tries to stamp this belief out of people, Hollywood's most successful creatives carry with them a strong belief that there is, eventually, some justice in entertainment, that talented people do eventually get ahead. "The cream rises to the top," I was told again and again, almost as if there is an official Hollywood handbook meted out that details which metaphors to use with aspiring writers to convince them that the problem is definitely them.

On the inside, I discovered a very different system. Talent agents weren't looking for talent, they were looking for dollar signs. They are, after all, professional salespeople. Sometimes talent and dollars are the same thing—a unique talent can certainly be worth money. There are a million other reasons those dollar signs can appear too, though, and a million more reasons that they can fail to appear even when a person has a unique talent. Seeing Hollywood's meritocracy's bubble burst wasn't as depressing as it sounds. It was useful. I learned how the system worked. Saw how successful people can game it. Stopped taking any slight or success as an indictment of my intelligence or my talent.

My experience with *The Village Voice* was kind of like that. I was, of course, depressed about our story being cut, but I also learned a lot about the reality of the news business, about what is and isn't considered newsworthy. It was a sales lesson. I saw that sensationalistic stories are what drive media on health and policy topics, not justice. That depressing realization can elude a true believer for years, but it's helpful to know.

With that said, the story's cancellation was certainly inconvenient. I had started the StuyHealth petition not because classmates were sick but because research had linked our exposures after 9/11 to health risks and our health care system made accessing care difficult and expensive. I didn't want us to get sick, an outcome that was nearly guaranteed, in a system where we couldn't get treatment. At the time, however, Stuyvesant students were, by and large, still young and healthy. All we could do was say that we expected to see these risks bear out over time, that help could not come after it was already too late, when we were already sick and underinsured. Compared to the really gruesome illnesses bubbling up in the responder community, however, the tale of an asthmatic twenty-two-year-old unable to afford her medicine or falling victim to preexisting-condition-coverage exclusions didn't quite do justice to the risks we were purporting to have undertaken. I could finally see that.

I took some other lessons from the *Voice* experience as well. Among them was that news outlets usually aren't interested in reporting on complicated tales of government malfeasance. Anything that has the potential to anger some of their most important insider sources, especially when it won't rise to the level of Pulitzer-genre trophy journalism, isn't worth the risk. We were putting a large public agency on blast and implicating every level of government, from the sitting New York City mayor to the sitting president.

I also hadn't known much about the culture of medical research and research funding when I undertook this project, and both turned out to be far more political than I expected. The media doesn't care about an issue you can't prove exists. The government doesn't spent money on hunches. For an everyday, regular citizen, however, getting data is nearly impossible. Data costs money. Money is power. Ergo, people without power are usually people without data. It's easy to overlook a population when you aren't gathering evidence on them, and that's sometimes by accident but also, sometimes, by design.

It's an old and wide-ranging problem—for years we've seen small news stories and quiet subheadlines illuminating the wide range of gender, racial, socioeconomic, and even political biases in medical research. In 1993 the US government attempted to address a major piece of the problem via the National Institutes of Health (NIH) Revitalization Act, which required that women and minorities be included in government-funded clinical health research.[152] The seemingly simple, obvious goal of including more diversity in health studies often fails to come to pass, even with that policy in place. Women, who are underrepresented in 9/11 health research, are also woefully underrepresented in broader categories of medical and especially pharmaceutical research. Drugs that cause disproportionate and sometimes dangerous side effects in women frequently make it to market anyway.[153] A vast majority of the drugs withdrawn from the US market between 1997 and 2000 were taken off the shelves due to side effects that occurred mostly or only in women,[154] meaning it took the suffering of women in the real world to prove that the initial trials were incomplete. Racial bias is also a big problem in many studies. In 2018 ProPublica found that in twenty-four of the thirty-one trials for cancer drugs approved by the FDA since 2015, fewer than 5 percent of the patients were Black despite the fact that African Americans make up 13.4 percent of the US population.[155] These absences lead to worse outcomes. Months into the COVID-19 pandemic we discovered that pulse oximeters—devices that measure blood oxygen levels and are a critical tool in the monitoring and treatment of COVID patients—were developed on non-diverse populations and are significantly more likely to give bad readings to people with darker skin. This leaves Black patients at higher risk for bad outcomes and worse care in a crisis that has already impacted them disproportionately.[156]

A lack of equitable data leaves activists in other advocacy fields with similar deficits as well. In 2020 the visibility of George Floyd's murder at the hands of police brought national focus to an issue police reform advocates had been talking about for years—that there's no standardized data on the incidence of use-of-force tactics by police. Without these statistics being tracked or reported, it's difficult to show governing bodies what communities of color have known for years from personal experience—that people of color, and specifically Black Americans, are much more likely to be the target of police violence than their white counterparts. This makes it easy for police departments and all levels of government to ignore the problem.[157]

Being represented in the data matters. At the most basic level, not having data means not having a credible story to report to media, it means not having numbers to back up your claim, it means not having facts to report to Congress about your mistreatment. It leaves people without a way to ask for help. This is why it's the sensationalistic stories that often break through to the public during community health crises and why, I realized, those would have to become our calling card too. The problem was, I didn't have a meaty sensationalistic story to offer.

Lombardi did fight for the story. A shorter version of it ultimately ran online on September 6, 2006. Not everybody Lombardi got on the record for the piece was happy to hear from us. Staten Island congressman Vito Fossella, one of the few Republicans working on the 9/11 health issue because of his district's large first responder population, said he hadn't heard about kids being impacted by 9/11. Then, inexplicably to me, he added, "Anyone who has been affected should state your case now. Or else."[158] Or else? Why it was necessary to give that angry warning is beyond me, especially given that his district was home to many Stuyvesant students at the time. It turns out, however, that being treated by members of Congress as opportunists instead of victims is par for the course. It's a rite of passage, one we got out of the way early. Naturally. Stuyvesant students are over-achievers, after all.

ON SEPTEMBER 20, STILL sitting in my father's office without much in the way of a to-do list, I got another press inquiry, this time from a reporter at the *New York Post*. The reporter, Elizabeth Wolff, was my age and had just graduated from Wesleyan along with several of my Stuyvesant classmates. I don't know how she initially heard about the petition, but I assume it was through the college-graduate grapevine. I once again sent out an email asking if anybody was sick or knew of a classmate who was sick and whether they'd be willing to speak to the press. This time I got a quick reply from a classmate named Amit Friedlander.

Amit and I had been friendly but not close in high school. He hadn't been very interested during the initial petition phase, though he had hesitantly added his name, probably more as a favor to me personally than out of any deep conviction. His email began with his noting that he hadn't really been following my updates, but it went on to say that this, in part, was because he had been diagnosed with Hodgkin's lymphoma in June and was undergoing chemotherapy. Though many 9/11-linked cancers have much longer latency periods, lymphomas were one of the earliest cancers to emerge in the 9/11-affected population, and Hodgkin's lymphoma was a cancer that a lot of first responders were already reporting. We had very little data, but we did have that fact.

Newly emerging after his initial treatment round, Amit was both willing to speak to the reporter and was newly radicalized on the issue. He was also primed for political battle, already planning to contact his elected officials and other media. Though he hadn't been following my middling efforts very carefully, he offered to work on the issue together. I put him in touch with Elizabeth immediately. Then, we started strategizing.

The story about Amit, which included a quote from me about the StuyHealth petition, ran in the *New York Post* on September 24, 2006. The *Post* often serves as a tip sheet for local TV news, so by the next evening Amit and I had also done a slew of TV and radio interviews and by the next day we were on the ten o'clock news on three networks as well as WBAI Radio. Reporters showed up at all hours, interviewing me on the noisy industrial street outside my parents' apartment. Trucks kept interrupting the audio. Lonnie, the owner of an antiques store downstairs and unofficial mayor of the block, smoked nearby so he could gawk and gossip with passing neighbors about what all the hubbub was about.

As is often the cycle in New York City local media, the TV appearances led to interviews in a couple of the local free dailies, *AM New York* and *Metro New York*. The headlines were sensationalistic, things like "Cancer Shock at Ground Zero HS," but most mentioned the petition, and we saw a sudden influx of interest from other advocates working on the issue, students who hadn't been reached by the initial petition round, and even some new naysayers who chastised us via Facebook or on the petition's website about taking attention away from responders. You're not winning if you don't have any naysayers.

In the days after the press bonanza, Amit and I arranged to get together and strategize, whatever that meant. We met on a park bench in Central Park, watching from just outside Sheep Meadow as Frisbee players darted back and forth, looking young, healthy, and collegiate. We chatted about the influx of press with wonder and some confusion. It had all happened very fast; then was over very fast. When we sat down, he warned me he had "chemo brain," that he had just come from treatment. I warned him that I had no idea what that meant. It was, unfortunately, not the last time I'd have to hear that warning from a fellow classmate. I'm now quite clear on what it means.

For somebody purporting to be a little out of it, Amit seemed very clearheaded. As the afternoon light began to fade and after-work sunbathers packed up their blankets and exited the park, he was still taking notes, making plans, breaking down my big, lofty ideas into actionable steps. We talked about other advocates we'd heard from, the talking points we'd use when speaking to them, about press strategy, about how to find out if there were other cancer cases among our classmates. We settled on nothing in particular, just the general agreement that we'd keep trucking along. Finally, he let me know he was too tired to keep talking and we parted ways, wandering out of the park in opposite directions. By the next day he'd sent me a detailed email with extensive notes from our chat. Amit is like that.

ON THE HEELS OF the press bubble, Scott Stringer's office called and suggested we seize on the momentum by organizing a press conference. This was a big step for us—it would not only announce that we were a constituency ready to be part of the discussion, but it would also get out the message to many new alumni that there was organizing to be done. The framing of the event was that we were going to thank the city for the $15 million in health funding that Mayor Bloomberg had just promised to use to expand an existing asthma clinic at Bellevue for downtown residents and anyone else ill from Ground Zero dust,[159] as well as encourage the federal government to pay their fair share.

Stringer's office invited both Congressman Jerrold Nadler and Council member Alan Gerson to attend—our two Stuyvesant alumni in office. They also invited some of the community advocates that I had not yet met. Amit and I, for our part, got a large group of our classmates to show up. We gathered behind a podium set up just outside of Stuyvesant. It was my first trip back to the school since this project had begun.

I'd been on a media whirlwind just days before, but the Stringer press conference was my first time ever giving an actual speech. I didn't have high hopes for my performance—I had long ago given up on my career in children's theater when it became clear that I don't actually enjoy being in front of people. (I was once cast as the "curtain" in a children's play because I was too nervous to improvise something on the first day of rehearsal. I've played trees more than once.) My nervousness had bled into my schoolwork in college. Raising my hand in class, which I'd done quite often previously, usually while simultaneously shouting out the answer, started to make me shake involuntarily. I became increasingly crippled by a subconscious layer of performance anxiety, and I began to avoid situations where I would be the center of attention. Then I stupidly decided I should spearhead an advocacy campaign.

To some extent, my sudden inability to handle public attention was par for the course. I've always been predisposed to developing new, arbitrary fears. When I was little, I was scared of nearly everything: dogs, the dark, bad grades, authority. You name it, I was nervous about it. Some of these fears went away, but most didn't. And I'd developed new ones since. Elevators. Cranes. Too much grass (hiding too many bugs).

The thing about being a perpetually nervous kid is that, because you get used to developing new anxieties out of the blue, you also get used to facing fears. A new fear of elevators doesn't mean you don't have to get home to the sixth floor somehow. A new fear of taxis doesn't make taking the subway at three in the morning any safer. Prior to 9/11, I became very scared of flying, but I like to go places, so at some point I decided to let myself be afraid of flying and get on planes anyway. For years, in order to have any quality of life, I've had to decide that my nerves aren't always worth capitulating to and that I have to just do stuff anyway. When my starring moment at that press conference arrived, I knew that I would hate it and that I had to do anyway. I shook all the way up to the mic, but I got there.

My speech was pure amateur hour. I read it off of the page instead of reciting it from memory. Having now stood in press conference crowds for many such speeches, I can say with confidence that reading a speech, rather than reciting it, is a great way to make boring remarks that don't deliver an emotive message. I'm sure that's exactly what I did, though a classmate standing behind me very kindly told me afterward that, though she'd been nervous when I took out the paper, she thought I somehow made it sound natural. I'm not sure I would have had the confidence to accept invitations to speak at future press conferences had she not said that. Her white lie gave me the confidence to try the public speaking thing enough times that I eventually got the hang of it.

I've delivered speeches many times over the years since. I still hate it— until the moment I'm in front of the microphone; then, I start to realize that it's not scary to be the center of attention when a cause is important. It's empowering and it's rare and it's worth basking in.

After the Stringer press conference, Amit and I were suddenly plugged into a much larger advocacy scene that included several local nonprofits, members of the downtown community board, and a group of Stuyvesant parents calling themselves the Concerned Stuyvesant Community. Most of these parents had been a part of the Parents' Association at the time of the WTC cleanup, and they had been plugging away for years to keep

Stuyvesant, whose students and faculty weren't well represented on the local community boards or in other neighborhood groups, a part of the discussion. They had a lively email list that, hilariously, included only one teacher—the one who had refused to write my SSR recommendation based on my activities in Cuba back in 2001. I hoped he didn't remember me.

Operating in the wilderness had been frustrating because it was hard to get our story out, but entering the larger 9/11 activist community had its challenges too. Most of the new interest in our petition and plans was helpful and supportive, but there was often a tinge of exasperation attached to it, always from older advocates who had been in the conversation longer. When Stuyvesant students began organizing, we didn't know enough about the political battles that were waged up until that point to know who wanted or needed credit for fighting them, so we hadn't given it in the press or in person. We were the youngest advocates by far, armed only with our own story. We had no in-depth knowledge of the issue's many political intricacies; we didn't know whose toes we were stepping on, just that we were often stepping on somebody's toes.

I'd known to expect some of this based on shadowing my mother through her many political lives. In any community of activists there are longstanding internal politics and longer-standing struggles regarding who gets credit. The reasons aren't necessarily petty, or ego-driven—credit determines who gets funding, who gets taken seriously by politicians and the powers that be, and therefore who gets heard. In our case, while most of the advocates were excited to have a new constituency step onto the 9/11 health scene, especially one filled with articulate spokespeople like the Stuyvesant alumni we'd been sending out on interviews, we were still widely perceived as late to the game. Other community members had been working on this issue for years; some of them were professionals by that point. They told stories of fighting the EPA early on, David-versus-Goliath-style confrontations with federal agencies, city officials, and others. They'd bird-dogged the EPA in the early 2000s over the agency's lies, periodically even driving them from their own events. They'd consulted experts in various environmental health subjects, become experts themselves, fought the cleanup battles as they happened, all while I was still in school. They knew a lot more than we did about the political history of the issue. And unsurprisingly, these advocates often took it upon themselves to point out to us in subtle and less than subtle ways that we didn't know what we were doing. It was sometimes frustrating, like having a thousand nitpicky parents monitoring your every move.

On the other hand, we absolutely did not know what we were doing. Still, our ignorance was probably more of a strength than it felt like at the time. We could say what we meant, even when we weren't supposed to. We could make mistakes that caused minor offense but opened up larger conversations that needed to be had. It was the freest I've ever felt to advocate for students without worrying about the political realities that constrain us and determine our success.

The idea that we were late to the game, however, still bothered me. We had been children during the attacks. The first year that anybody who had been a minor on 9/11 was old enough to be out of college and spearheading this kind of project was 2006. We didn't owe something to the activists who'd spoken up on our behalf before. They were just doing what was right—protecting kids—and now so were we.

This, of course, is something I can say in retrospect. In reality, there's a time and place for deference. Amit and I learned pretty quickly that being an effective advocate involves more than just speaking up about a cause— you need to have good people skills too. As soon as we finished our second big press tour of the week, we dove headfirst into connecting with as many advocates as we could and educating ourselves about some of the struggles we had missed. Amit reached out to members of the downtown community board and tried to get up-to-date regarding the Bellevue clinic that was seeing a small group of Lower Manhattan residents. I, meanwhile, met with a few of the parents involved in Concerned Stuyvesant Community

(CSC), who gave me a helpful rundown of what the school's parents had been up to while I was not yet of drinking age.

The first thing I learned was that Concerned Stuyvesant Community's organizers had something really important that we didn't—a paper trail. They had access to documentation detailing the Stuyvesant air quality battles, as well as intel about where the small amount of government funding going to the 9/11 community was coming from, the likely outcomes of the various lawsuits that were working their way through the courts, and the local movement's different players. One member of the CSC was working with an organization called 9/11 Environmental Action and put me in touch with their director, Kimberly Flynn. That seemingly casual referral changed StuyHealth's trajectory immensely—Kimberly and 9/11 Environmental Action, both critical parts of the early efforts to protect the residents of Lower Manhattan after 9/11, became a vital source of support for StuyHealth's work in the following months and have remained so.

The Stuyvesant parents were generous with their time and information, but they were also dismayed that their work had not been highlighted in any of the coverage Amit and the petition had gotten. They felt like they were being left out of the loop politically now that staffers at the offices of Borough President Stringer, Representative Maloney, and Representative Nadler were getting in touch with me, and sensitively noted that they shared the primary concern that people seemed to have about us—that our petition demanded something big and distracting: health care for life. The conversation everybody else was having by that point was focused on smaller, more achievable goals geared toward the community that was still living downtown.

Amit and I diverged a bit in terms of how seriously to take these kinds of comments. I maintained that it was not a bad thing for somebody to come bumbling in with a big ask. Big asks risk distracting and annoying people working in the policy weeds, but they can restart larger discussions that have died on the vine. When you've been working on an issue for a long time and are living in the minutia of negotiations with entities that aren't interested in helping you or admitting what they did wrong, you can lose sight of what true justice even looks like. What we offered was a broad perspective, perhaps, but it was an important and unique one as well. Amit, on the other hand, wanted to prioritize realistic goals. Of course he did—he was sick.

The bigger issue with joining the community in asking for local services, I argued, was that many of us were not local. A group of Stuyvesant alumni were still living in the neighborhood, but thousands of us were in the process of creating adult lives elsewhere or would be in the next few years. We both were and weren't a part of the neighborhood, and that was something that needed to be clarified, even if the initial response from other activists and politicos framed us as naive. A clinic in downtown Manhattan doesn't help anybody living in Oregon. Or Washington. Or Texas. Or Illinois. By late 2006, many of our classmates lived three thousand miles from downtown Manhattan.

Knowing where our needs differed from the community's helped us find our voice. We stopped talking solely about wanting health care for life, but we kept our talking points focused on the fact that we were geographically dispersed—something we had more in common with the rapidly organizing first responders than the rest of the downtown community. Our perspective filled a void, and soon it became clear, even to people who were annoyed by our unintentional showboating, that we had something to add.

PERIODICALLY MY MOTHER CALLS me up and says, "I'm having an idea day," then rattles off four unrelated new plans or goals, all of which require emails and calls and research on my part. She drops them in my lap like they're weightless, like a free idea costs nothing in brain space. I'm usually enthusiastic at first, excited about the possibilities. As I gather my thoughts, I start to refute the new plans she's pitching one by one, not because they aren't good ideas but because there are only twenty-four hours in the day and the one thing I have plenty of already is good ideas. I, too, like to think of myself as somebody who is good at hatching big ideas. What I don't have are good execution skills. That's where I often need help.

In mid-December I came to Amit with one of my big ideas—a student lobbying trip to DC to educate members of Congress about the needs of the young adults in the 9/11 community, especially since many former students were now living in other states. He was in, in so quickly that I was startled. Suddenly I was left with the challenge of actually making it happen. The very quandary my mother is always getting me into, now self-imposed.

On the federal level there wasn't much coordination going on between the two House offices working on 9/11 health legislation, so the most complicated part of this "big idea" was in deciding whether to support Representative Nadler's bill or Representative Maloney's bill. Given our relationship with Nadler's office and his status as an alumnus, we decided to support his plan, the 9/11 Comprehensive Health Benefits Act of 2006, which would have coordinated 9/11 responder and survivor care through Medicare and the Veterans Administration.[160] The bill's appeal for us, as a rapidly dispersing population, was that the proposed health program would be run through large public programs that operated nationally. The health program established in Maloney's competing bill, the Remember 9/11 Health Act, would have contracted with private insurers to provide care at specific locations,[161] a more worrisome plan because it might be inaccessible to classmates outside New York and also because it threatened to add more private insurance battles to our already overwhelming pre-ACA plate. Insurance concerns aside, however, our choice pitted us on a more complicated side of the political battle. As staffers from numerous offices warned us, Mayor Bloomberg, and therefore New York's City Hall, supported Maloney's bill.

As I began working on the details of the lobbying trip with an interested group (ideas might require only one person, but execution is a team sport), we continued to receive alarming reports of illnesses in the Stuyvesant community. Amit got an email about one classmate's battle with an aggressive ovarian cyst, which her doctor had said could be a precursor to cancer. In mid-January he forwarded me an email from his mother. It was an appeal for bone marrow donors for a Stuyvesant alumnus with an aggressive form of leukemia. He was a few years younger than us, and the email was from his aunt, who had sent it to the student body at a different city school. It read:

> Sam was a student at Stuyvesant on 9/11—which the family speculates may have led to his illness. He was one of hundreds of kids who, upon seeing the towers collapse that day, headed home covered in dust from head to toe. He was supposed to graduate from Harvard this spring. Now he is dying at a New York (Cornell) hospital and is in desperate need of a matching bone marrow donor.[162]

Because his ethnic background made it difficult to find a bone marrow match, Sam's family was sending the appeal wide in hopes that somebody with similar heritage would step forward—he was biracial: half Asian, half white. We learned that there were very few Asian marrow donors in the system, let alone any that would be a good match. Sam was already quite ill, so we made a cursory attempt to get in touch with his family but didn't want to generate any new obligations for them. Still, this was the second Stuyvesant student to be diagnosed with a cancer similar to the ones first responders were reporting, both cancers appearing within only a few years of the attacks and in a very young cohort. We were spooked. I tried to forward the email around to the 9/11 health advocates, but almost all of them said that they were no longer sending match requests out to their email lists because they came too regularly.

By January, reporters and other advocates were frequently asking whether Sen. Hillary Clinton, who was taking the lead on the 9/11 health issue in the Senate, had responded to our petition. Only a few days after our press conference in October, she'd fired off a letter to Alan Steinberg, the EPA's regional administrator, asking for a "comprehensive testing and cleanup program" for Lower Manhattan.[163] The letter referenced Stuyvesant's case specifically. Soon after, one of her aides got in touch with me and updated me about the legislative situation on the Senate side, which was good intel for our planned lobbying trip, though it kept getting pushed.

The competing bills in the House made coordinating with the Senate side a little complicated, but all parties appeared at a January 22 press conference organized by Representative Maloney, as did both Senator Schumer and Senator Clinton.[164] The presser was held just before President Bush's State of the Union address, and the demand, according to the press advisory the offices emailed out, was that President Bush "include medical funding for 9/11 health monitoring and treatment in this year's federal budget and finally come up with a plan to medically monitor anyone exposed to the toxins of Ground Zero and treat everyone who is sick."[165] Somebody in Maloney's office loved wordy sentences.

The crowd was to include a group of 9/11 responders whom Senators Schumer and Clinton and Representatives Maloney, Nadler, and Hinchey had given their State of the Union gallery passes to. I got an email announcing it from one of Representative Maloney's staffers, and I assumed I'd be attending just to stand around in the background of the live shot and look concerned (a classic part of the political theater experience). Then, a few days before January 22, I learned that I was being invited to speak as well. This time I was not only speaking in front of Representatives Nadler and Maloney, by now not a big deal for me, but also in front of Sen. Hillary Clinton, that era's (okay, every era's) most famous woman in politics. It was especially high-pressure because she'd announced her intention to run for president just two days earlier, meaning the press turnout at the event was massive.[166]

January 22 wasn't the first time I'd met Hillary Clinton, but it was the first time that I met her in a meaningful context. Prior to that day I'd shaken her hand once, in the fall of my freshman year of college. That year there was a gubernatorial election being held in New York. A new friend and I had taken a trip down to the city to poke around and take photos, the hobby I had adopted as a way to make friends. During our wandering we happened to run into Hillary Clinton on a street corner downtown—she was campaigning for one of the candidates, Carl McCall. Instead of taking a picture with her, I took a picture of her and my friend. It just seemed like my friend wanted the moment more. She loved celebrity, loved identifying famous people in the wild. I played the part of the hardened New Yorker, unimpressed by everything. I regret being so blasé. Not because it would have made my day that year but because, though I've met Hillary Clinton many times in the intervening years, there is no photographic evidence that we've ever crossed paths aside from a couple of wire photos of that January 22 event, all of which show only the very top of my head. Short person problems, I guess.

There was also some action at that January press conference. Nobody knows this, but for a brief moment I was an unsung American hero. That's because while everybody else stood around looking concerned, embroiled in the theater of the presser, I was called upon to act as Senator Clinton's human shield.

Because she had served as First Lady, Clinton traveled with Secret Service protection. As we gathered in front of the cameras, two guys in suits and earpieces stood off to the side flanking the gathered advocates. As we had first congregated, a woman holding a poster and shouting something nobody could understand had been standing off to the side. People yelling random, potentially crazy things on the street is peak New York. Nobody batted an eye. As the crowd for the press conference formed, however, the shouting lady's interest was clearly piqued. Slowly she made her way into the huddle of advocates gathered behind the podium, and at some point, Clinton's aide leaned over to me and said, "Don't move—there's a crazy lady behind you. But it's okay—the Secret Service is right there."

Another advocate and I closed ranks around the senator so that the woman wouldn't have a clear view of her, and I nervously looked to see where exactly the Secret Service was. Apparently "right there" was Secret Service code for "miles away, largely irrelevant." They could not have been any farther from us without exiting the event altogether. We stood stiffly, trying not to look over our shoulders, not actually tall enough to block the view of Clinton's head, until the woman finally wandered away. I think I can definitely say that I saved a life that day.

The distraction of a crazy lady working her way into the crowd was helpful on some level—it gave me something to focus on besides the speech I was about to give. As is always the case for the nonresponder advocates, I was scheduled late in the lineup, and the long road to the podium was otherwise occupied with quiet knee stretches and a slowly blossoming backache. When I finally did speak, I once again read from a paper. By this point I had at least figured out how to look up for long stretches and make brief eye contact with reporters in the crowd. The reporter field was notably thinner than it had been during Clinton's remarks.

Still, though Senator Schumer left right after his remarks (a frequent move of his), Senator Clinton stayed through the end, and as I passed her on my way back from the podium, she patted me on the shoulder and said a distinct "Good job." Clinton and I have had our political differences over the many years of her public service, but I can honestly say that as a young female advocate just learning her way around the world of public speaking, I have never been more excited to hear that from anyone.

UNLIKE THE YEAR IT followed, 2007 had momentum from the get-go. In February, just about a year after I had sat down to write the StuyHealth petition, I got my first almost-honor. Scott Stringer's office was hosting a State of the Borough speech, a hilariously local event ambitiously modeled on the State of the Union address. The speech is generally a way for the borough president to highlight the issues their office has been working on all year and introduce the local players. Amit and I learned in early February that we were going to get a mention, during which we'd get to stand up and wave to our adoring public. It was held in the city council chambers, and we attended along with a who's who of that year's community advocates, which is to say, nobody we knew or recognized. I spent most of the speech mesmerized by a large crack running down the wall of the otherwise spotless city council chambers. In a city government notable for its unsavory connections to the real estate industry, that seemed like a meaningful metaphor for something. I'm still not sure what.

Still, the event was a nice way to commemorate how far our work had come. It was also motivating. I didn't know back then how rarely people who do advocacy or community work get their efforts noticed or honored. The story of being a survivor advocate is, essentially, seeing benefit events focused on 9/11 health all over the news and social media, then noticing that they don't even mention nonresponders. Having a government official give a speech in a stately room and say that our efforts mattered was important and helpful as we continued to organize our classmates.

A couple of weeks later, in early March, we finally made our lobbying trip to DC as well. The plans had been in continual flux for several months, periodically overheating my logistics brain. The March trip very nearly got canceled too, due mostly to the chaos of the congressional schedule. Nadler's staffers were overwhelmed, their priorities shifted hourly, and the constant postponements were nothing we could predict or problem-solve our way around. It took a panicky evening phone call to Representative Nadler's chief of staff, who was definitely in the middle of making dinner and very kindly took my call on her cell phone, to finalize the date and strategy. With my brain a puddle on the floor but a date finally set, I reached out to the pool of students who had expressed interest in joining back when the trip was scheduled for January. I tried to sound like I had some command of what was going on. I didn't.

Four students, including Amit, ultimately agreed to meet me down there, fewer than had initially shown interest—but a miracle nonetheless. One was an alum I barely knew, another a good friend of mine from my Stuyvesant days. He was in school nearby and provided a steady stream of positive reinforcement as I pretended my way around. Then there was a tangential friend who had discovered an interest in activism and shit-stirring in college—a bit of a wild card, but she was funny and periodically, through her stoned-looking stare, said something so apt and articulate it would pull everybody back to the point. She brought a drooping backpack and was dressed like she was planning to hang out on a street corner and skateboard later. To be fair, I hadn't accumulated much in the way of professional wear either. I was in continual denial about the bit of weight I'd gained in college, which made it difficult to buy properly fitting clothes. Either way, I was pleased to hear that anybody at all was available. Then, a second miracle occurred. Kristen Lombardi, *The Village Voice* reporter, agreed to join us on the trip.

We took the Hill by storm on March 8, by which I mean I led an army of four twentysomethings and a reporter through the doors of the Rayburn House Office Building. We gathered in Nadler's office, got our meeting schedule, and were set loose on the Capitol. Lombardi noted, as I led the group into the tunnels that connect the House office buildings and toward our first meetings, that I seemed to have a strong command of the Hill's layout. I'd like to say it was thanks to my superior civics education, but it was all thanks to my mom. Everybody should be so lucky.

My mother used to lead tours of Capitol Hill for the Close Up Foundation, an organization that takes kids around Washington to teach them about civics and government.[167] That's how she learned the ins and outs of the House and Senate office buildings, and when I was a kid, she made sure I learned my way around them too. If I expressed surprise that regular citizens can just walk into our representatives' offices, a comment frequently made by the uninitiated, my mother would act like I was being ridiculous.

"The American people own these buildings," she'd say. "We own them." I should be clear that the implication was not that we should act disrespectfully. She was definitely never suggesting that I endanger the lives or safety of the public servants who work there for us, as pro-Trump insurrectionists would do on January 6, 2021, using a similar line of reasoning.[168] She just wanted to make it clear that I shouldn't ever deign to worry that I didn't belong on the Hill. That as an American, I was personally invested in the activities of Congress, and that I should focus instead on getting more out of my investment.

Every casual trip to Washington we ever made included a trip to the Capitol, but sometimes we went to DC for protests too. In 1998, my mother let me skip school so we could attend a protest in DC on the eve of the Clinton impeachment vote. A few of the Judiciary Committee's impeachment hearing celebrities, congresspersons like Rep. Maxine Waters and Rep. Jerrold Nadler, were holding a rally outside the Capitol. We were grumpy—we'd come down on a bus at five in the morning with a group of the loudest, most incessantly chatty people we'd ever encountered, so we'd gotten no sleep, and President Clinton had just decided to bomb Iraq,[169] something we absolutely did not support. We rallied for a while, then wandered off. In our wanderings, we stopped by the office of a conservative New York congressman, the representative for the upstate district in which my parents had bought their first home and have voted on and off for years. Much to our surprise, we were told he would meet with us personally.

The meeting went . . . terribly. My mother questioned his support for the Clinton impeachment, and he quickly grew enraged and began shouting. He talked over us. He mansplained sexual assault to us.

It wasn't exactly shaping up to be an inspirational story about democracy. That meeting was, in fact, a little scary. I don't remember specifically how my mother responded to him because I was already in fight-or-flight mode, but I do remember watching her body language change as he hovered over us. The contrast between them was extreme. My mother, as I've mentioned, is

4'10"and was seated on the arm of a chair, shrinking her further. The congressman must have been at least six feet tall—but while I cowered at his aggressive congressional finger-jabbing by shrinking, my mother got angry. She marshaled the force she'd used as a teacher in the New York City public schools and argued right back. In the midst of the chaos, she demanded from a powerful man that he respect the most sacred tenet of democratic government: that our representatives work for us. That whether or not he agreed with us, it was her turn to talk. Then she marched us out of his office. We exited on our schedule, not his.

After that experience, walking into Congress just to take some decorum-filled meetings felt like no big deal. I was new to single-issue lobbying, but I could say with confidence to Kristen Lombardi that, yes, I knew my way around. As the other Stuyvesant alumni we were traveling with marveled at how easy it was to get in, I used my mother's favorite line: "Of course it is. We own these buildings."

THERE'S A LOT MORE to know about the Hill than just geography, of course. Our March 2007 lobbying trip was a major learning experience for me not just in the art of advocating for legislation, which the entire group and I were terrible at, but also in how to read the mood and intentions of a congressional office and interpret their advice. Being on the Hill can be a little disillusioning, especially when you're there to talk about a serious issue that impacts you personally. I spent large parts of the day fighting to keep my head up as we struck out in various offices.

In school you make some assumptions about how government works. You assume that being a politician involves a lot of going to hearings (it does), but you don't realize how often the hearings are empty. You assume that writing legislation involves hearty debates among dedicated and good-hearted public servants (it does), but you don't realize how often the choice to support or ignore that legislation is more about PR strategy than justice.

Depending on where you are from and how straight your congressperson's office is willing to be with you (a lot of New York offices pride themselves on their straight talk), you don't realize how much more leverage giant financial interests have than you do when it comes to getting bills passed. Those are all things you learn in your first few days of lobbying, but there is still something uniquely empowering about being on the ground.

Capitol Hill is flawed, of course, but for a regular American citizen, there is something gratifying about experiencing, firsthand, the piece of your civics curriculum that teaches you that you have the right to go into any congressional office and say your piece. You do not need a special pass or special permission to tell your elected officials how to better serve you. Balancing that feeling of power with the feeling of disappointment that government doesn't always work the way it should is key. That morning in March was rough, but by the end of the day we were all feeling at least some of the power that comes from telling the people who can truly change things that they should, in fact, change them.

Most of our meetings were on the House side, but we did meet with Senator Clinton's office early in the day to debrief about the battle on the Senate side. They told us about a hearing that would take place on March 21 at which Michael Bloomberg would testify and invited us to submit written testimony. The request was without much conviction—Amit even wondered aloud later whether they were just giving us an activity to be polite—but they did note that the chair of the Senate Committee on Health, Education, Labor & Pensions (also known as the Senate HELP Committee) seemed to be on board with doing something for our community. Clinton's office was already assuming that the best-case scenario was a program that would need to be renewed every five years, and their short-term goal was to get members of the HELP committee who represented districts outside of New York to actually show up at the hearing. I had no idea what a Herculean task that was at the time—I'd spent much of my childhood watching hearings with my mother, who thrived on the subtle theater of them, but only the hearings that made it to television. Those were usually the high-impact ones that people wanted to show up for. I didn't realize then that most hearings are essentially held to put stuff on the record, a record that nobody ever consults anyway. Bringing Bloomberg in was an attempt to draw some eyeballs, but it was a long shot despite his celebrity. He'd likely be testifying to a largely empty panel.

On the House side, meanwhile, we spent much of the day trying to figure out where offices stood in regard to the Nadler/Maloney two-bill drama. Offices varied in their reaction to our choice to support Nadler's bill, a choice I quickly realized we shouldn't have had to make. One of the unspoken rules of lobbying is that you are supposed to be there in support of a bill or a specific policy. Offices don't want to just meet with you to chat; they want you to have a clear, actionable ask for them. We had an ask, and thought that in choosing the bill that would better serve our specific subset of the affected community, we were doing the best we could under the circumstances. Instead we fielded a lot of frustration and even anger from offices that were supporting Maloney's bill, or an unwillingness to engage in the situation from offices that didn't want to cross the two New York cosponsors—both of whom were relatively senior members on important committees. We were set loose in a jungle with arbitrary rules. It hampered our ability to share what we needed to about the needs of the young adult community.

As we walked between offices, I played the series of events that led us there over and over in my head to keep myself motivated: The federal government had knowingly exposed us to dangerous toxins as kids, then chastised us for coming to the battle late, then given us two pieces of already agreed-upon legislation to choose from, only to tell us that the choice had infomally already been made by the time we got there. Repeating this time-line over and over served me in the same way that my doctor's warnings about the danger of the air downtown had. I remembered the facts so as to remain impervious to half-truths and deflections. I used that internal monologue to guide me as I led our tiny army into battle.

We met early in the day with staff from Rep. Vito Fossella's office, the Staten Island congressman who had given Lombardi that bizarre quote about how people should state their case now if they wanted help "or else." His office said they were working with Representative Maloney on reopening the 9/11 Victim Compensation Fund, a pot of money the federal government had set aside for victims' families that would later be expanded to cover the illnesses and deaths of 9/11 responders and community members,[170] and expected legislation to be introduced that month. At the time we didn't really understand what that had to do with us—the original Victim Compensation Fund was for those who had suffered harm on 9/11 and for the families of those lost during the attacks.[171] It hadn't served the survivor community, and Fossella's office didn't seem to know or care if they'd changed that. They were very focused on responder needs, on being patriotic and using the word "hero," on framing the response to 9/11 as something akin to a military action. They didn't seem to know that there were other layers of need in their district. We did our best to point out that we had classmates who'd lived there. They heard us in the technical sense, but not in a meaningful way.

After Fossella's office we met with the office of Rep. John Hall (D-NY). Hall was an upstate New York representative who was most famous for being a musician in the seventies. His office had a subtle hippie vibe, and they gave us an early win by adding his name to the cosponsor list on the Nadler bill immediately. It was the highlight of the day. Staffers for Rep. John Tierney (D-MA) were polite but disinterested. I had insisted on stopping by the office of Rep. Kirsten Gillibrand (D-NY) because she represented the district whose angry impeachment-era congressman my mother and I had faced down in 1998. My grandparents still lived there, and I knew that there were 9/11 survivors living in the area as well. They hadn't heard much about the issue and were mostly curious if anybody was cosponsoring both bills since, as a freshman office, they didn't want to get in the middle of an in-fight. We could relate.

Gillibrand's staffer reiterated that tying the issue to a representative's district is key, but I also remember asking the staffer if she was from the district—they'd just had major floods in one area, and I was going to ask if she or her family had been affected. She replied that she was from Florida and was looking forward to visiting the district for the first time soon. One of the more fascinating parts of visiting Capitol Hill offices is learning how few staffers are from the district they work for or even passingly connected to it.

One office that didn't share that "we'd love to see the district one day" vibe was that of the powerful Chairman of the Ways and Means Committee, Rep. Charlie Rangel. Rangel (D-NY) was a longtime power broker from the New York City delegation whose office was staffed by older, no-nonsense aides, not the fresh-faced twenty-somethings we'd been speaking to everywhere else. Many of them had clearly been with Rangel for a very long time, and almost all were New Yorkers themselves or had at least developed the right accent in the intervening years. Rangel's staff didn't beat around the bush with us—they told us that Nadler hadn't been pushing hard with them for his bill and that they were following the lead of Bloomberg's office, who had told them not to support it. They somewhat patronizingly cautioned us against asking for cosponsorships on a bill before developing enough political support for a cause—a classic Hill holding tactic—but they were the only office to get into a truly substantive back-and-forth with us about possible funding mechanisms. It felt like even when we disagreed, they were taking the meeting seriously. Halfway through, Representative Rangel wandered through the room and we were introduced to him, one of the only times we got to meet an actual congressperson that day.

Rangel's office did, in passing, say one other thing that surprised me— that while there was a lot of political pressure to do something about this issue, nobody in their district had ever notified the office that they were a 9/11 survivor. As if, after years of being assured that the government had definitely not put them in harm's way, constituents would think to call their congressman's office with a quick health update. Still, because of the lack of outcry, 9/11 health issues weren't being viewed as a true constituent concern beyond their role as a broadly New York-associated problem. That's why Rangel's office was letting Nadler and Maloney take the lead. We jumped in on that point and noted that there were Stuyvesant alums who came from their district, some of us in that meeting, in fact, so they could no longer say this. Certainly their district didn't have damage on the scale of Nadler's community, but this was, in fact, a constituent issue.

According to Amit's notes from the day, one last thing that came up with Rangel's office was the idea that dog and other animal disease statistics might be useful indicators for future health issues in people since animals often get sick quicker than humans. I don't remember this exchange, but I'm not surprised we brought it up. The idea had been stuck in my mind for years. Even up in Chelsea, about three miles away from the World Trade Center, every dog in my parents' building had died of an oddly virulent cancer, some suspiciously young, within five years of 2001. This stat, about five dogs total, included my childhood dog, Noah, who passed away while I was in college after developing a strange, fast-growing tumor. Within two years every other dog in the building was gone too. I've heard people from other neighborhoods talk about this as well, but nobody ever did those animal studies. I think if they had, they'd likely have discovered that the health consequences of 9/11 were much more widespread than the federal health programs addressed—that people living far uptown and in outer boroughs beyond Brooklyn were also breathing in dangerous amounts of WTC dust. The fact that the only office that ever discussed that idea with us represented a district so far uptown (Rangel's district was north of Nadler's and covered most of upper Manhattan) was interesting.

There were many ways in which that trip to DC was valuable to me personally and to the people I traveled with, but the most beneficial outcome was really about optics. The trip made clear that we were an engaged cohort, so both Nadler's and Maloney's offices began to keep us in the loop. In mid-March, about a week after the trip, Maloney's office called me about an updated version of their bill and even solicited my thoughts. I took their request seriously and sent them a lengthy reply that highlighted a couple of concerns.

The legislation was an updated version of their plan, which involved having the federal government pay for care for survivors as a secondary insurer. True to my brand, my first comment was something big—so big that many other members of the community hadn't even considered it or thought it would be too obvious to mention. Nobody can see the flaws in the health care system as clearly as somebody who has just started to navigate it for the first time. Essentially, I was concerned about the idea of using private insurance as a basis for the 9/11 health services the government would establish. Rangel's office had given us a hint about why the law might have been written that way—nobody wanted to establish a precedent that meant that any group with a claim like ours would have to be added to the Medicare system. Given how much support there was for adding everybody on earth to the Medicare system in the 2020 election cycle, at least in Democratic politics,[172] it blows my mind that this flirtation with the Medicare system was the holdup. To me, using private insurance contractors to coordinate the services meant that companies whose entire purpose is to avoid as many costs as possible—companies I'd been personally fighting with growing exasperation as I tried to figure out how to cover the cost of my asthma medicine—would be in charge of health services for traumatized people.

The bill had a shiny silver lining, though. Students were explicitly mentioned for inclusion in everything from the health services the bill would establish to the committees that would guide those programs.[173] Despite the promises of the New York congressional offices, our inclusion in the federal response to 9/11's health crisis was never a guarantee. Just a month earlier, on February 28, the Department of Health and Human Services had held a hearing about the impacts of 9/11 that, according to later testimony from Representative Nadler, indicated they "had no intention of including area residents, workers, and schoolchildren in the plan they are ostensibly developing to provide care to victims of post-9/11 environmental contamination."[174] Being named in the legislation mattered.

Looking back on those emails is a little exciting—I was young and inexperienced, but I had obviously taken great care to give thoughtful and thorough notes. A sign that I was still pretty new at this stuff, though? My email font at the time was Comic Sans. You live and you learn.

ON MARCH 21 I headed back down to Washington for the hearings Senator Clinton's office had mentioned. Concerned Stuyvesant Community kindly offered to pay for Amit's and my share of a rental car so we could drive down with a couple of other advocates. (Luckily nobody asked us to get behind the wheel. Nobody should ever ask a native New Yorker to get behind the wheel. We don't know how to drive.)

The hearing was scheduled to start at 10:00 a.m., so we left New York around four in the morning, hyped up on caffeine. I talked for all five hours of the trip about entirely forgettable things. I'm the kind of nightmare of a human being who would do that. I selfishly reasoned that somebody had to keep the driver awake and we were all excited to be on an adventure, so we made it work. There were other talkers in the car too. Amit was rightfully exhausted by us nearly immediately and dozed on and off as we motormouthed.

The hearing room seated about four hundred, and a decent-size crowd was milling around when we arrived. As Clinton's office had teased, however, many hearings aren't necessarily attended by the committee. A couple of senators wandered in and out, but for the most part the witnesses spoke to an empty line of chairs presided over by Senator Clinton.

The experience had a surreal quality, in part because I was tired—I'd woken up at three in the morning—but it was also my first live hearing after what I've sometimes described to friends as a very "hearing-forward" childhood. It was like getting to visit the set of *Mister Rogers' Neighborhood* or some other childhood classic television show. I eagerly basked in watching the actors up close, seeing the set pieces with my own eyes, observing the pageantry behind the stoicism. Like Hollywood, Washington is a good place to work if you're kind of a ham, and there's something a little charming (although sometimes deeply concerning) about that. For every boring five-minute presentation in a hearing, there's a hilarious, two-minute, flowery, honorific-filled introduction of a person nobody likes whom somebody has to find a nice way to introduce to the crowd anyway.

After we sat through hours of introductions and comments, the group meandered over to a nearby room, where Senator Clinton's office had planned a press conference to follow. Though we wouldn't be speaking, we were told we should approach the press after the main remarks while everybody was set free to wander around glad-handing. In reality all we did was loiter in the background of the huddle, speak to nobody since nobody knew who we were, and leave. Five hours back without much to show for it, and I probably talked the whole way in that direction too.

Things slowed down a bit after that hearing, and despite all of the excitement of that fall and winter, I was, at the end of the day, still a marginally employed college graduate with no real idea what I was doing with my life. There wasn't any money in working on 9/11 health issues—I'd done the whole thing on the cheap using free blogging platforms and donated transportation. I didn't want to spend my time fundraising. I wanted to stop working at the dusty nonprofit where I was stuffing envelopes part-time for a pitiable wage, and while I didn't want to go find a full-time envelope-stuffing job, I did dream of one day moving out of my parents' house.

With no idea what else to do, I waded back into my regular life—the one where I'd wanted to write for a living—and in May I signed a short-term lease in Venice, California. The move taught me a lot, as big moves generally do, but leaving New York proffered me one lesson in particular that I wasn't prepared for: there is no way to "check out" of a major traumatic experience.

CHAPTER 8

A MODERN NETWORK

I had been offered a couple of jobs in politics by the time I moved to California in May 2007. I'd turned them all down. Instead, I set off on a last-minute, minimally planned road trip across the country because being twenty-three is like that sometimes. I told my parents that it was a temporary, easily reversible decision—that I didn't want to regret not trying something, *something*, with my life. I couldn't articulate what that *something* might entail, but the word "townie" had wormed its way into my brain and so I blamed my trek out west on not wanting to be one of those. After all, though nobody calls New Yorkers townies, we're as susceptible to sheltering ourselves in familiar surrounds as anybody else. Just because those surrounds include upmarket sushi and famous art museums doesn't make them any less familiar.

The logic behind moving so far away was mystifying to my parents. To some extent it still is. They were incredibly proud of my work over the previous year and didn't understand why I wouldn't take the clear win and get a job out of all the effort I'd put in. What was the point otherwise? They were simultaneously, however, very eager to get me out of the house, not so much because I was cramping their style but because they came of age at a time when people could afford to rent studios in New York City on entry-level salaries. They often worried aloud that my continued presence in their apartment was a sign that I wasn't making mature choices. In a runaway real estate economy. With no job. In retrospect, adorable.

Internally, my view on the California matter was much hazier than what I projected, but that was part of its appeal. I wasn't that committed to the state itself; I knew almost nothing about what awaited me there, but though the move was one part lark, it was also one part clandestine effort to switch paths professionally before the rest of my life got steamrollered by 9/11. The pressure I was facing from every corner of my life to pack it in, move to DC, take a job on some congressional staff, absorb 9/11 into my professional identity, and dismiss my other ambitions as the naive objectives of an optimistic kid with no respect for the rules was astounding. My insistence on Los Angeles was meant to be so out of character and bizarre that it reset everybody's expectations. It was going to be a terrible fit for a high-strung, fast-talking and -walking New Yorker, and that was, in many ways, why it was the perfect place for me. I made plans to crash at a high school friend's house until my short-term rental was ready and to forget about 9/11 for a little while. Beyond that, nothing.

THE DRIVE TO LA was long. Too long. For over a week my high school friend Nina and I argued about the merits of country music for eight-hour stretches as we precariously drove a hand-me-down yellow VW Beetle with a manual transmission through the flatlands of flyover country.

It was an outlandish premise. Two native New Yorkers, two terrible drivers, setting out alone to see all the parts of the country we'd been warned about. We'd stuffed the car with the makings of an iconic road trip—a trunk full of toiletries and clothes, a cooler filled with oranges, a GPS machine so heavy that it would rocket off the dashboard at random intervals, and a finicky portable CD player connected via cord to the car's tape deck. We made stops at Graceland, swooped into Louisville on the day of the Kentucky Derby, saw the Petrified National Forest, the Grand Canyon, and friends from college we thought we'd never see again because they'd moved so far into the middle. Sometimes we stayed with those friends; sometimes we showed up at hotels and asked if they had any rooms free as if it were still 1970—before cell phones, when people could still be spontaneous about travel.

In Duck, West Virginia, we named the car "Ducky" because of its physical similarities to a rubber duck. In Arkansas we almost got struck by lightning (I felt the metallic taste in my mouth as a bolt struck the tree next to us). In Norman, Oklahoma, we panicked over a tornado warning, then almost got stuck in a flood. We laid low in Texas because our dads had given us holdover advice from the sixties about how much Texans hated New Yorkers and hippies. In Flagstaff, Arizona, we got into a fight about whether we should see the Grand Canyon at dawn or during regular daylight hours.

We found ourselves continually flabbergasted by how big everything was no matter where we were. As we ate at our first Chili's, we marveled at the size of the sodas they served and the fact that they would refill your cup before you'd even half-finished the first pour. We saw sky of a size that didn't seem real and trains so long they defied logic. By the end of it, Nina had finally learned to drive stick, I never wanted to see the inside of that car again, and we made it safely to the land of In-N-Out, Los Angeles, California, where I'd spend the next fifteen years of my life seeing basically only the inside of that car.

On the day that we arrived in Marina del Rey and first slept on my friend's smelly college-era couch, I could still have recited the chain of events that leads from one bad high school grade to a life of ruin. I tossed and turned, starving after making the unfortunate discovery that I don't actually like In-N-Out burgers and exhausted from the drive, trying not to rest my nose near the vomit-scented couch cushions. I sat with the dull awareness that I was, essentially, choosing to proactively ruin my life so that the ruin could be a foregone conclusion instead of a hammer that might fall at any moment. I didn't really care. After rehashing terrible memories for public consumption for over a year, I needed a little time to be idealistic and idiosyncratic instead of practical. I continued to feel the pressure of the DC life beckoning, however, especially as my friends from high school made their way there one by one and quietly settled down.

As far as why I didn't want to work in politics, that's an argument that's still evolving, a battle I'm still fighting. For one thing, I don't think anybody should be obligated to have their professional life tie into the worst day of their life. Advocating as a constituent is empowering because it's a choice—you aren't required to think about 9/11 all day, every day. Within the context of a career, however, where the obligations are less flexible, less self-determined, and more all-consuming, working on 9/11 issues would be more like a slow-rolling torture.

Beyond my hesitancy to absorb 9/11 into any more of my life, to allow it more space than a hobby, there were also tangible, brass-tacks, fundamentally solid reasons that I didn't want to work in politics in general. Unfortunately, the only one that I could articulate to people that summer was that I didn't want to wear a suit, as if I was uniquely offended by them, as if other people love putting on a structured, uncomfortable outfit every morning with an unnecessary noose-like accessory, slipping into the stiffest of leather shoes, and heading out the door.

In retrospect, I see it was the rigid environment that a suit projects that was the problem, not the clothing itself. The getup was a lightning rod. Harping on the outfit was just my youthful, inarticulate way of describing that I didn't think I'd flourish in "that kind" of office job. I was drifting through the closing years of an investment banking bonanza that siphoned off smart kids, paid them zillions of dollars, then robbed them of their youth by sitting them at desks for eighteen hours a day and making them look at spreadsheets. "That kind" of office job was a popular choice since it offered prestige and security. I understand why people were excited to have those things. Having spent the year arguing that my classmates and I were failed by many of those seemingly secure structures, however, I saw the stability of those prestige jobs as false and fragile. I couldn't make myself believe the sacrifices that they would entail would be worth it. For one thing, I saw my good health as potentially fleeting, and for another, who knew if those secure jobs would be there in two years anyway?

I also found it hard to articulate my feelings about the moral trade-offs that working in politics requires. Nobody is supposed to talk about that part of public service because it is, by and large, an admirable profession that requires some praiseworthy sacrifices. Still, every person who works in politics must, at some point, make a trade-off between their personal agency and their professional needs. Today, after well over a decade of advocacy work, I am more confident than ever that my personal agency—the fact that I have spent years advocating for myself and my classmates in a relatively uncomplicated way, saying the things I believe without worrying about career-ruining professional pushback—is the one thing that has kept my mental health intact as I talk ad nauseam about the government imperiling my health and recite the events of the scariest day of my life. That's not to say that there haven't been many stretches during which I've felt the tug of people yanking my agency away so that my presence would serve their needs. It's more that, through those experiences, I've always had just enough independence and freedom to say no to their demands when they crossed a moral line.

Working in politics, even working for "the right side," requires you to give some aspect of your constituent power up—you cease to be a meaningful voter when you work in the politician's office. Once actual constituent needs become a problem for you to solve instead of an issue for you to raise, your priorities, by necessity, have to change. We saw it all the time in the 9/11 health world. People who I know personally *wanted* the survivor community to have benefits equal to those of responders got put in the position of explaining to us why it was logical that we *didn't* have them. Better for the cause. Fair. Every interaction with a staffer was laden with this subtext:

Of course you should have these things. Unfortunately, getting them is impossible. Instead, let me explain to you why it's actually better for everybody. Don't worry, I'm good at my job. The thing is, most of them were good at their jobs. Still, it requires a strong constitution to handle that kind of routine disappointment, and, if I'm being frank, I'm the opposite of thick-skinned. I cried a lot as a kid. I'm easily startled and upset. I find it physically painful to deliver bad news to people. I think there is a perception that being a good advocate requires being impervious to criticism and unusually tough. What it requires instead is simply caring deeply about an issue, enough so that you're willing to be uncomfortable from time to time. Working in a political office itself, however, requires an armor I don't come by naturally and certainly could not have faked in my early twenties.

These days I'd go even further and say that my interest in politics is, in fact, rooted in my independence from it as a profession. There have been times that I've had to rely on political work for money and times where I've had to consider the political implications of the funding I've received because every funding source, even when well meaning, has its own baggage and priorities. Overall, I like being a constituent and an activist, and I don't particularly like being beholden to mundane considerations about how to make a living in a way that aligns with my principles. For me, that ruins a little bit of the magic, though many people have argued to me that being on the inside gives you a different, more powerful kind of agency. Often, however, the pro-"inside" people don't know what it's like to work on the "outside." You can achieve meaningful victories out here too.

It was not until the heyday of the Occupy movement, years later in 2011, that I finally figured out how to articulate all of this. Occupy Wall Street started in New York's Zuccotti Park as a protest of rising income inequality, inspired by the Arab Spring and sparked by a group of local activists and the Canadian magazine *Adbusters*,[175] but it grew into something much broader than that—a wide-ranging, leaderless, left-wing movement that espoused many of the progressive left's concerns about capitalism, police violence, corruption, the environment, and more. That movement was constantly derided for being disorganized and lacking clear demands,[176] but to me that seemed like part of its unique power. Protesters were asked to come and offer what they could, not what central organizers demanded.[177] Those who were good at organizing made connections between activists instead of decisions about how their volunteer labor would be used. Those who were artists set up creative public art projects that reflected the many reasons people showed up to fight. Those who liked to cook set up impromptu kitchens in Zuccotti Park and other parks across America and fed the protesters. Writers volunteered to write. Computer geeks volunteered to livestream. Nobody was asked to stuff envelopes.

I loved this about Occupy. It was a new kind of movement, one built on a messy, sometimes complicated consensus that gave people the ability to decide where they could best contribute, then trusted them to do the work. For years people said that Occupy accomplished nothing, but I disagree. It did exactly what it intended to—it raised the issue of growing income inequality (among other issues), and it changed the language we use to discuss both the problem and potential solutions. It also changed the protest tactics that movements use to engage people, and it did so without asking anybody to waste hours of their life completing a boring task to which they were poorly suited.

What I took away from watching Occupy operate was that the process of determining how to be effective on a political issue should involve some self-reflection. It should involve trusting that you know your talents better than anybody else. Organizations, for their part, should encourage you to be proactive with those talents. For some people, being given a helpful process-oriented task list is plenty. I've heard lots of people tell me they find stuffing envelopes meditative. I don't. I find it maddening. On the political end, many find working within the political system and negotiating complicated compromises rewarding. My closest childhood friend is a genius at navigating these processes, and I've often been jealous of her skill set. It's incredibly valuable. I don't have it.

Before Occupy, at age twenty-three, I didn't have the language or leverage to say outright that working toward somebody else's political goals, for a politician I wasn't fully aligned with politically, or for an organization whose focus was necessarily compromised by its fundraising obligations, wasn't going to serve me or them. Instead, I bailed out of the conversation. I moved three thousand miles away from my opportunities and started over. Being in your twenties is like that sometimes. I did ultimately realize, however, that what I was doing was choosing to trust myself, choosing to see where my talents lay, and choosing to participate in the ways I knew I could be helpful. I was electing to retain some agency over how my labor would be used, to what political ends my time would be harnessed. I was electing to be a partner, not an envelope stuffer. It was the only setup that made political involvement tolerable to me, and as somebody who was raised to take my civic responsibilities very seriously, I knew I had to find a compromise that would.

I'm a hypocrite, of course. When I left politics behind I went to work in Hollywood, another industry that requires unsavory moral trade-offs. Aside from the suit thing, it's actually pretty similar to the Beltway. Still, when Hollywood is corrupt, the scale of the destruction is different. Nobody in Hollywood has ever made a snap decision that's resulted in the deaths of thousands of Kurds or stopped millions of people from having access to clean water. Slimy executives have famously made reprehensible personal decisions, of course, but professionally their decisions, at most, have the power to desensitize us to acts of violence or normalize bad behavior. They don't have the power to make us complicit in their badness. They can't fund violence on the scale that Washington can. In Washington, politicians and their teams hold millions of lives in their hands. They have the power to fully shift our reality, not just our perception. The stakes are a little higher when you sell out in politics.

I WAS STILL PRE-HOLLYWOOD in my first California summer in 2007, of course. Pre-career of any sort. I missed some important events in Washington while biking around Venice Beach and taking calls from the boardwalk, but for a while, I didn't care. When Representative Nadler's office held hearings that spring, I submitted written testimony, and in September 2007, Representatives Maloney, Nadler, and Fossella introduced the 9/11 Health and Compensation Act, which would provide comprehensive medical coverage and health monitoring for anyone—not just first responders and volunteers but also the survivor community composed of office workers, residents, and students—who were exposed to the dust at Ground Zero. It also called for the reopening of the September 11th Victim Compensation Fund, which, having already paid out claims to the families of the victims of the attack, would be repurposed to provide financial compensation to sick and dying 9/11 responders and community members.[178] I experienced light FOMO, but still toyed with the idea of dropping the issue altogether now that I'd said my piece. In our advocacy world, survivors dropped the ball and walked away all the time. Many of the advocates who have stuck with the cause since the beginning were not there for the attacks themselves; they were simply a part of the community in the aftermath. For those of us who experienced trauma on September 11, and even more so for people who got caught in the dust cloud, it can take a lot of mental fortitude to stick with work that reminds you every day of the scariest moments of your life. Most people eventually burn out, and I figured I could be "most people."

Being so far also away gave me some perspective on why I shouldn't give up, however. It showed me how many gaps there were in the 9/11 health story the rest of the country was hearing, how few people understood the full scale of the problem. As responders got sicker and, consequently, more organized, I watched nonresponder survivors struggle without a similar sense of unity and community. Just like people in California didn't know who we were, *we* didn't know who we were. Our organizations were still trying to determine the boundaries marking where our survivor group began and ended and how to find representatives for constituencies like mine, victims emerging years later, scattered throughout the nation. Having spent the year taking stock of my memories from that time and learning the details of the Stuyvesant cleanup (or lack thereof), I realized that just my store of knowledge alone was a valuable asset—few people with insight into the unique needs of the exposed kids and young adults were on the scene. I felt responsible, and if I'm being honest, I've never quite felt relieved of that responsibility. Even in moments when there have been more voices than just my own speaking for the young, it's become clear to me that community activism is a "more the merrier" kind of situation. I remained tethered, engaged almost against my will, still struggling with a vague need to find a real life too.

Many of the conversations toward the end of 2007 and into the beginning of 2008 were about research and pediatric treatment protocols, boring things about science that were, unfortunately, really important. I slowly picked up the necessary medical terminology—I'd often find myself Googling scientific terms from the desks of various temp jobs. I spent days reading up on comorbidities while covering for the receptionist at the Tennis Channel and researching pulmonary conditions while answering the phones at Merv Griffin's real estate firm. When I eventually got a gig as a script coordinator on a television series, I thought I'd finally transitioned into my new life and could look forward to a long, rewarding career in television during which I'd make zillions of dollars writing and retire in my late fifties, complaining about how nobody values *experience* in Hollywood. Instead, the Writers Guild went on strike and I began working at a promotional agency and in freelance production, struggling to find traction and watching my future and career spin away from me. Through all of it I would go home at night, check my email, and talk about health care and environmental exposures, because 9/11 was the one consistent thing I had left. I could not freelance my way away from it.

In February 2008 a funding opportunity came up through the Health & Hospitals Corporation (HHC), and StuyHealth began to officially collaborate with 9/11 Environmental Action, the Kimberly Flynn–led nonprofit that worked with the Lower Manhattan community. The funding covered a very small, very part-time salary for me and some of StuyHealth's web and outreach expenses. In exchange, I did outreach work online to students and schools from the area with information about a new 9/11 health program located in New York City, an HHC clinic treating survivor patients at Bellevue Hospital.[179] The bulk of the grant went to 9/11 Environmental Action, which did the same outreach (with much more success) to residents and area workers. The health program didn't offer much to students outside New York, but having a program to point community members to was better than nothing.

It was an interesting time to begin collaborating officially with the other survivor groups. The larger activist community's go-to tools for communication had changed between 2001 and 2008, and it felt like there was a huge schism between younger activists and their older counterparts. The schism wasn't caused by the usual things—differing places in the economy, different experiences, different wars. It was caused by social media. A lot of what StuyHealth was attempting to do by existing online had no parallel on the ground with the more traditional community groups. In fact, it had no parallel anywhere aside from with other young people working on other causes. It made me seem like an expert in something, but, frankly, I had no idea what I was doing most of the time—there were not exactly best practices to follow for engaging an audience on Facebook yet. The ways in which we were all seeking to create social ties on the internet were new, and the reasons it would end up being a challenge to have meaningful conversations online weren't well understood enough back then for us to troubleshoot them.

One of the differences I noticed right away between how the online and on-the-ground outreach groups operated had to do with how we used imagery. I quickly became very conscious about using upsetting copy and pictures from 9/11 itself in online outreach. It was too easy for people to quickly click away from pages that brought up bad memories and never seek out more information. Deciding to focus on positive messaging and imagery was a major shift—a lot of the informational outreach to the 9/11 community in that era used pictures of dust and destruction. Visual reminders of September 11—images of people (even children) covered in debris, the towers collapsing, the broken steel girders of Ground Zero—were pro forma. While working with 9/11 EA, I slowly began moving toward more upbeat messaging. I wrote copy about things you could get for free paired with generic cityscapes and stock images of doctors. It felt a bit like a catch-22—how does one sell information about illness and trauma but make it look fun?

I also began writing about the topic and sending out essays on health care and 9/11 survivors to any editor of any online section or paper that I could scrounge up an email for. My first op-ed was published by *The Guardian* and ran in an online opinion section called "Comment Is Free," on the anniversary of September 11 in 2008. My "comment" wasn't "free" to them because they paid me (unheard of!), but that essay also allowed me to put into words the primary frustration I had with how rhetoric about 9/11 was being used on the national level and specifically in that year's presidential election:

> As a 9/11 victim and part-time community organizer, I know that the memory of this event does have a place in this election. But, instead of being used as a rationale for the continuing "war on terror," as an excuse for decimating the Bill of Rights, or a segue into a discussion about the "successes" of our war abroad, the events of 9/11 should prompt a conversation about this government's failed health policies. That conversation should not be limited to 9/11 alone but must include other national disasters like Katrina. Instead, any discussion of these disasters, man-made and natural, provides the basis for

the argument that America needs a health care plan that covers everybody. Now.[180]

THE BIZARRE CHOICE TO describe myself as a "part-time community organizer" might have been so distracting that nobody could see beyond it, but the larger point was one I've tried to make whenever possible over the years—that health care, or our lack thereof, is the one thing we have in common with every other disaster victim regardless of whether the disaster is man-made or natural, big or small, accidental or intentional.

For years I continued to write essays for *The Guardian* whenever I had a burst of anger about the way 9/11 was being discussed or used, the way 9/11 victims were being ignored, or, sometimes, just the way my generation was being battered by a bad economy. I started writing for the *Huffington Post* as well, expanding to any source that would give me a platform, because not only did I want our story elevated, I wanted to use 9/11 to elevate other disaster victims too. 9/11 survivors have a lot in common with the victims of other acts of mass violence, of environmental injustice, of climate change. At times we've shied away from making those connections because our political system leaves us all fighting for funding scraps, but the parallels are powerful. There's strength in those numbers too. After the BP oil spill in the Gulf in 2010, I wrote:

> 9/11 and the BP oil spill may not have much in common in their details, but they will likely have a lot in common in the coming years. Even President Obama has compared the magnitude of the spill to our experience with 9/11. Just as is the case with 9/11, there will inevitably be long-term consequences to this oil spill that we can't predict or even imagine. Who will be responsible for covering those ongoing costs? Will it be BP? The US government? Or, as we see with victims of 9/11, will the people of the Gulf have to fight tooth and nail to get what

they deserve in compensation for years to come? The heroes of 9/11, after all, still have no long-term commitment to care from the federal government.[181]

As for my own long-term care, in 2009 I became a patient at the World Trade Center Environmental Health Center (WTC EHC) at Bellevue, the New York–based program we'd been doing outreach for on our HHC grant. After years of stockpiling medicine and carefully doling out half doses, I'd calculated that it was literally cheaper to fly to New York for my asthma care and medicine, which was free at the WTC EHC, than it was to get the care near my home in California and pay the copays on the visits and medicines. Exhausting and not very efficient, sure, but much, much cheaper. I tacked on screening appointments to trips back east and alongside family time, stops at my favorite food spots, and long walks with my close friends, I began to spend a few hours of every visit to New York waiting in line at the Bellevue pharmacy. When Advair is saving your life, you do what you have to do.

BEYOND MY DAZZLING SUCCESS in *The Guardian*'s opinion pages, 2010 wound up being an important year for the 9/11 community for other reasons as well. In the first few years of my involvement in 9/11 health advocacy, we'd seen small bursts of funding go toward programs like the survivor clinic at Bellevue and several disparate responder services, but there had been little action on the 9/11 Health and Compensation Act, the health bill first introduced in 2007, then reintroduced as the James Zadroga 9/11 Health and Compensation Act in 2009 by Rep. Carolyn Maloney in the House and Sen. Kirsten Gillibrand in the Senate. The bill was similar to Representative Maloney's original 2004 proposal, but unlike that legislation, the 2009 Zadroga Act was supported by the entire New York delegation (finally bringing an end the era of warring House bills).

It called for $3.5 billion for the establishment of the World Trade Center Health Program, a federally funded monitoring and treatment program for responders and community members, as well as $4.2 billion to expand the criteria for the Victim Compensation Fund.[182] Though I'd supported Representative Nadler's proposal in the two-bill era and this iteration of the 9/11 health program proposal hadn't been my first choice, it was now our only choice.

The Zadroga Act didn't even get out of committee in 2009, and unfortunately, 2010 didn't begin on a promising note. At a meeting in January, Health and Human Services Secretary Kathleen Sibelius announced that the Obama administration would not be supporting the bill.[183] In February, facing some blowback from politicians and activists, the White House proposed doubling the level of federal funding going to the existing 9/11 health programs,[184] a paltry offer compared to the scale of the need. In September, with midterm elections coming up and a Republican sweep looking more and more likely, Obama finally decided he would support the Zadroga Act.[185] With a thumbs-up from the White House, the end of 2010 looked like it might be our last chance to pass the bill for several years. A GOP midterm sweep was looking likely in the House, meaning the chances of the Democratic-led legislation even getting a vote in the next Congress would fall to below zero. We had a small window to work with.

As I floated between my freelance production gigs that year and tried to figure out my career, I also began to hear more about new cancers among classmates and other survivors, as well as the seemingly ubiquitous chronic illnesses that were afflicting the 9/11 community. In the summer, just after I wrote the op-ed about the BP spill, I brought up some trivia at a dinner party with high school friends.

"Did you know that acid reflux is one of the most common conditions seen in 9/11 responders?"

My friends looked around the room and agreed that they hadn't heard that. They also, however, agreed on something else—that every person at the table had a fairly painful, serious version of acid reflux. We were all in our mid-twenties, all otherwise healthy. It was not a good omen. Acid reflux/GERD is not the sexiest disease to bring up at the dinner table, nor the most serious sounding. It is, however, incredibly expensive to treat once it becomes serious and chronic. It also increases your risk for other complications and even esophageal cancer down the line.[186] The medicine I was being prescribed for it at the time cost $150 a month and I was only making about $22,000 a year. Fortunately, once I joined the Bellevue program, the cost of the medicine was covered, but I was the only person at the table signed up for that program. Looking at how quickly responders had moved from minor chronic conditions to cancer, I worried about what this bout of widespread minor illness meant for us down the line.

AFTER MY MOVE TO California, I'd been carefully choosing when to engage in 9/11-related work, sometimes attending meetings back East, sometimes dropping in on phone calls, but 2010 was a hard year for me to ignore the 9/11 conversation. After a sudden rash of deaths struck my close family beginning in the spring, taking an aunt, an uncle, a great-uncle, and both of my maternal grandparents, and I wound up back on the East Coast for much of the year, stuck in the thick of the advocacy scene whether I wanted to be or not. Because I'd been very close to my grandparents, I was designated to be my grandfather's caretaker in the summer following my grandmother's passing and spent several months traveling between upstate New York and New York City. He died of a stroke that fall, but before he did, and despite the sadness enveloping everything around us, we had a ball. We had long-winded, esoteric arguments, not with the intent of disagreeing, but to develop our talking points, and then we'd pepper the people around us with seemingly outrageous ideas. He would sometimes channel his sadness into bizarre, funny declarations. He famously announced that phones were at the center of our nation's ills during one car trip through town, and, when asked to expand, declared, "They're making it too easy to communicate." We spent a lot of time watching long, ponderous sports—contemplative events like marathons and cross-country races followed by macho, fast-moving sports like football as a palate cleanser. He suffered from advanced macular degeneration, so he could barely see and I cooked and helped him with household tasks, then took him on long, slow walks through town. I left in early August, after which my parents took over feeding him and keeping him company. I rushed back just a couple of days before his passing in early October, eager to get to his bedside as hospice took over his care.

After the trauma of that year, my family was in crisis. Everybody was in shock, nobody was getting along, nobody could figure out who should take the piano but half of us weren't ready to talk about the piano yet and the other half were really, *really* concerned about what to do with it, as well as the other mountains of stuff at my grandparents' house. I was able to develop such a close relationship with my grandparents because my mother had one. Now my mother was coming apart at the seams. I stayed again, this time to take care of her.

Thanks to those tragic duties, I was in New York when the campaign to pass the Zadroga Act kicked into high gear that fall. Responder groups had been hitting the halls on the House side since 2009 and were by then a well-oiled machine. After the White House changed its tune in September, the Democratic-controlled House quickly passed the bill and sent it on to the Senate.[187] Things did not move as quickly there. A lot of legislation was being held up by a new Republican innovation—the repeated and aggressive use of the filibuster. Bill opponents weren't standing up and talking for sixteen hours about Dr. Seuss or their favorite recipes or whatever Mr. Smith did in *Mr. Smith Goes to Washington*,[188] but every piece of legislation required a cloture vote, meaning every bill needed sixty votes to even get to the floor. The Democrats had had exactly sixty members in the Senate until the death of Ted Kennedy in February 2010, when Republican senator Scott

Brown won the special election to fill the seat.[189] The forty-one Republicans had been holding strong in filibustering any new spending bills, no matter how important, for months since. At times, some of the more conservative Democrats joined them. Even in the sixty-vote-margin era, we had watched a Democrat, Sen. Ben Nelson of Nebraska, kill the public option in the original Affordable Care Act debate.[190] Needless to say, the 9/11 advocacy focus switched immediately to the momentous task of pressuring the Senate to act before the end of the year.

In October, as I looked for a cellist to play at my grandparents' memorial, I got word that I could tag along to DC on a Senate lobbying trip with the FealGood Foundation, a first responder organization run by a mouthy ex–iron worker who had lost part of his foot during the 9/11 rescue efforts.[191] I sensed that John Feal's level of influence was admired—not without a trace of jealousy—by other 9/11 health advocates. He was an instinctive, gifted organizer—he could generate hundreds of calls to DC from sick and angry cops, firemen, and construction workers with a simple email. He was bombastic and larger-than-life, unafraid to dress down a politician and, periodically, unafraid to dress down his own guys.

I'd known John for years, though, if I'm being honest, I couldn't always tell if he knew me. We had been introduced many times, and would often find ourselves in the same meeting or standing in the same presser crowd, but our organizations hadn't really interacted beyond friendly hellos. His relationship with the larger survivor community was touch and go. The careful, meticulous, detail-obsessed survivor advocates sometimes found his uncontrolled brand of machismo-fueled indignation confusing and threatening. They were working at two strategy extremes.

Despite periodic trips to DC during which I'd tack on congressional walk-throughs, I hadn't been on a true lobbying trip since 2007, so I said yes to the FealGood Foundation plan without hesitation.

The Senate in 2010 was wild and frustrating and a little squirrely, but there was another layer of complication too. Hillary Clinton, the Senate lead on the bill, had just left to work in the Obama administration.[192] Her replacement, Sen. Kirsten Gillibrand, had been appointed only months before and was still getting up to speed.[193] She was a congressperson (one we'd lobbied back in 2007) from upstate New York who had big shoes to fill on this issue and no track record to speak of when it came to 9/11 and health care. The last thing we needed in what was already a tiny window for victory was a new variable.

ON THE MORNING OF October 28, I waited in front of the Senate offices to meet the FealGood Foundation. Given that I had arrived in DC sick from stress, exhausted, and in mourning, it seemed appropriate when I saw what appeared to be the guests of a Mafia funeral approaching. The hoard of men in black suits filtered out of their bus slowly, ponderously, and began, in waves, to cross the street. They looked a lot spiffier than I expected. I had evidently missed the memo about dressing professionally, which must have come with the memo about having your reading materials prepared and remembering to be over six feet tall.

A member of the first wave smiled as he approached, eight other huge men in tow. "Yes, it's us." He broke into a wide, goofy grin that I had to look straight up to see.

The strategy session began almost immediately. We were split into groups and directed to certain offices at specific times. We had a folder with all of the information we needed and a keeper of the folder, a group leader of sorts. My group also contained a number reader, who told each Senate office how many first responders had come from their state and how many were sick.

As my group began to wander toward our first meeting, the "Mayor"— real name Ron Jones, a New Jersey politician with a fondness for discussing his friendship with New Jersey governor-elect Chris Christie—introduced himself. His nickname was literal. He was the mayor of a small town, one I had never heard of but that was in an area where many of the men and women who had worked in the Twin Towers had lived. Our other two group members were responders, one an NYPD chaplain and one a man who'd been nothing more than a concerned citizen volunteer and had gotten a brain tumor because of it.

The Mayor asked me who I was, the odd woman out. He wasn't really asking who I was at that moment. The answer would have been complicated. "Failed TV writer." "Perennial production assistant." "Coffee gopher." "Person without any grandparents." He was asking who I *was*. What I had been on September 10, 2001. I said my piece: that I was a high school student at one of the first schools to return to Ground Zero; that I had been back in Lower Manhattan by October 9, 2001. I discussed breathing in the smoke from the fires and the dust from the debris barge located next to our building, attending school in a neighborhood that had become a National Guard–led state, looking out the window in every class to find a skyline suffused with smoke, and missing its most prominent feature. Unlike the rest of the lobbying group, of course, I hadn't volunteered. I was seventeen. The city sent me there.

Again and again, I've been the person who tells this kind of first responder—tough, job-hardened, a lobbying professional—about the kids of 9/11 for the first time. Most responders weren't from the Lower Manhattan community so they didn't see any of this happening or, if they did, had bigger fish to fry at the moment. At the end of the story it's always our lack of agency that gets them. The first responders were deservingly called heroes because they had stepped up in a moment of great national need. I had been volunteered by forces beyond my control. I had nothing heroic to show for it aside from my presence. Luckily, that was enough for them. We made our rounds.

If I'm being honest, I also had an ulterior motive for joining the October DC lobbying trip. I was in my twenties and so FOMO-filled after watching the excitement of the Obama inauguration from California that I'd promised myself I'd make it back east for the next big thing. "The next big thing," if you were somebody my age, was the Rally to Restore Sanity and/or Fear, an event organized by Jon Stewart and Stephen Colbert to comment on how bizarre and ridiculous the nation's political culture had become. It happened to fall on the same week as the FealGood Foundation's lobbying trip, and it was the rally that finally gave me the excuse to bite the bullet and commit to both events with the purchase of a nonrefundable bus ticket. I needed to support the 9/11 community, but I also needed something fun to mark the end of a horrible, death-filled, family-drama-ridden year.

That rally was, incidentally, just a couple months before Jon Stewart invited a group of first responders onto his program, *The Daily Show*, and became irrevocably associated with the 9/11 health issue. I doubt he even knew we were down there with him. He had tens of thousands of fans to joke around with, a televised event to put on. I watched him from among a sea of thousands, craning my neck just to see a sliver of his face on a jumbotron three sections deep into the crowd. I figured that was the closest I'd ever get.

ON DECEMBER 9, 2010, the Zadroga Act was finally introduced on the Senate side but defeated in a cloture vote.[194] On December 16, 2010, Jon Stewart invited four responders onto his show.[195] He'd done a segment on the bill back in August and had been growing increasingly furious about the Senate's inability to get it passed, especially since politicians had invoked 9/11 to justify so many other expensive policies. He wanted to put the focus squarely on the people whom the Senate was turning its back on, so a group of four responders I'd seen around the Hill and at New York events were given a chance to make a pitch directly to the American people. The publicity their appearance generated created a huge amount of public pressure on the Senate to do something.

The swift change was heartening. Jon Stewart was, by this point, very aware of what his platform offered to a cause like ours and was committed to using it in a way that was meaningful. It was, at the same time, one of the more cynical political lessons I took from that year—that having a celebrity advocate your cause, no matter how worthy it is to begin with, is one of the few ways to it get noticed. I had long wondered why seemingly random celebrities are often invited to testify before Congress on issues like women's health—topics they are perhaps committed to but are certainly not experts on. I never wondered again. The celebrity publicity machine, when it can be harnessed for good, is incredibly powerful. Stewart not only interviewed responders and personalized the 9/11 health story during the December 16 telecast, but he also called out the major news networks for failing to report on the Zadroga Act's progress (or lack thereof). The next day those networks, major players like CBS and ABC, reported on Jon Stewart's charges and, in the process, began to cover the Zadroga Act too.[196] Soon it was a major national news story.[197] Within days, resistance in the Senate began to dissipate. We had a window, but no promise of a vote.

IN LATE DECEMBER, I headed down to DC again on a FealGood Foundation bus that left at four in the morning from a desolate, snowy corner near Penn Station. My mother walked me there, her presence further inflaming speculation about how young I was. A couple of guys I knew from the last trip promised her I'd be taken care of, a promise I was grateful for as I stepped onto the bus to realize I was one of only two women, and certainly the youngest by at least a decade. That had predictable consequences. The responder I sat next to talked the entire way down, just about general stuff, his thoughts on politics, on the inconveniences in his life, on his 9/11-related illnesses. His monologue didn't stop when we arrived in DC. He followed me around for most of the day. Eventually I was taken aside by the one female responder and cautioned not to give him my personal information; he'd been repeatedly contacting her by phone long after she'd asked him to stop. I was finally removed from his company by a phalanx of other responders who noticed what was going on and thought his interest had become a little too forceful. They were right, and I was grateful for their intervention. Those bodyguards are friends of mine to this day. That man? Somebody I've avoided on many trips since.

The rushed timing of the end-of-year lobbying also presented its own oddities—many senators were either already home for the holidays or plotting their escape, so we met with staffers in jeans who were ready to show us the door the moment we arrived. The Republicans knew they'd be in the majority in the next term, but we begged them to consider a vote before the end of the year so the final bill would have time to be approved by the House. Rumors flew about what offices were making what demands, and finally it became clear that our only opportunity to get the bill done would be to cede to a demand from two of the Republican members on the fence, one of whom had been a medical doctor in a past life (of course). Sen. Tom Coburn of Oklahoma, half of the hold-up, was so famous for stopping legislation that his nickname in the Senate was "Dr. No."[198] He and Sen. Mike Enzi of Wyoming, the ranking member of the Senate HELP Committee, wanted a cheaper bill.[199] The Zadroga Act's funding period was cut down from ten years to five. Finally, they said okay.

I can't say I personally had much agency over the last-minute negotiations with Coburn and Enzi. Gillibrand's staffers, John Feal, and others did the dirty work. I never even got to meet the men. I do, however, remember the offices of the senators we lobbied that day, all Republican members from midwestern and southern states. They felt much vaster and more unconquerable than they had on past visits. Many were packed with hunting-themed paraphernalia and imagery in ornate golden frames. Images of violence. Five years of funding was an outcome we'd been prepared for, but as we walked the halls we marveled at the heartlessness of their hard-liner stances and the crocodile tears of their staffers as they essentially told us, "We won't help you." Tom Coburn later passed away of prostate cancer, one of the most common cancers among the responders he met with and tried to block five years of care to. He was only seventy-two, relatively young, but older than a lot of the 9/11 victims he saw on that visit lived to be.[200]

A final vote on the five-year bill took place on December 22, and we watched from the House and Senate galleries as it passed. In the House gallery we were told to remain silent but cheered anyway when the bill got enough "yeas" and, for a moment, it felt as if the floor of the House turned into the British House of Parliament, with both members and gallery observers stomping and cheering. In the Senate we nearly missed the moment because the bill was passed via unanimous consent quickly and quietly. It wasn't until Sen. Chuck Schumer gave us a thumbs-up that we realized we'd won. A federally funded health program was on its way, one that offered much broader care than the small local programs we'd been relying on.

To the community's great relief, the bill that passed included a category for "survivors," the people living, working, and attending school near Ground Zero.[201] Such an inclusion wasn't guaranteed—I didn't realize until after the fact how close we were to being cut out of the programs entirely. I think I was being purposely naive, unwilling to acknowledge many perils of the DC legislative process unless absolutely necessary. I should have probably known as much, though. We regularly faced this threat, sometimes by other advocates, sometimes by the very people charged with negotiating for these programs on our behalf. Sometimes even, in moments of pure desperation and frustration, by the very offices that introduced the bill. I always assumed these were empty threats, more theater than substance. I was wrong.

The survivor community was, and remains, a touchy subject for a few reasons. The biggest one is our size. After the air was declared safe to breathe by the federal government, hundreds of thousands of people returned to live, work, or attend school in the disaster zone.[202] (Hundreds of thousands of likely deserving people were ultimately cut out by the bill's arbitrary geographical boundaries, of course. A lot of survivor advocates still get calls from sick people outside the boundaries who have credible concerns about 9/11-related illnesses.) By any estimation, the cost of doing the right thing for that community, because of its larger size, is much greater than the cost of covering care for the roughly one hundred thousand first responders[203] who breathed in that same air and did their lifesaving work beside us. There are, to put it simply, many, many more of us.

There was also the fact that, since we were rarely at the forefront in news coverage, we were vulnerable in cost-cutting discussions. We knew ahead of time that fiscally strict Republicans would likely demand concessions. We saw what the Jon Stewart publicity had done for responders, but we didn't have a celebrity mouthpiece. Our situation was complicated and required context. We couldn't generate enough public interest to protect us from being a concession.

Our inclusion also had the power to set a significant precedent. It was our chance to get an admission from the government that it had a responsibility for what had happened to the community. An admission was key to keeping us in the conversation in future funding rounds but might allow other communities to make similarly expensive claims to government services. Charlie Rangel's office had told us this was a risk in no uncertain terms back in 2007.

Despite my naivety about how close our funding was to getting cut, I had started to play defense. At some point in late 2010, I realized that I was not really there to tell the student story to congressional offices directly. Sure, I'd been doing it on and off for years and they would contort their faces into looks of concern or sadness when I described being a kid on 9/11 and having to go back to school, but none of them had heard much about our community before, knew the extent of what we'd been through, or particularly cared about a bunch of mostly non-constituent New Yorkers and ex–New Yorkers. My real role was to share that story with responders in front of congressional staffers so that they could react, repeat the story, and get it heard.

Lobbying is a bit like improv; you have to "yes, and" the situation sometimes. You have to listen. You have to pay attention to where your openings are. I was always the youngest 9/11 advocate walking the halls, but I faced an additional invisibility issue stemming, let's be honest, from my gender. Everywhere we lobbied, there was an unspoken sense that the 9/11 health issue was really about men. The media focus made it seem like all victims were first responders and all first responders were men, so that was who the nation saw as the affected population. In meetings, even when female responders came down with us (there were, of course, thousands of female responders), the focus was always on men's health and traditionally male-dominated jobs and qualities that we associate with masculinity, things like heroic rescues that relied on strength and power and the ability to dominate physical obstacles. Because of this, being heard often meant finding a man who would repeat my story to the people who could actually change things. That, after all, was when they were most open to listening. I don't love admitting that, but that's improv. You have to work with what you're given.

Though it certainly wasn't ideal, the strategy proved effective in our context. Responders had separate health programs and their own priorities at this time, which meant that sometimes the downtown community didn't feel very welcome when it came to their meetings and their events. The guys in my FealGood lobbying groups were always surprised when it turned out that there was something really complementary about the stories we were telling. They'd start off skeptical, but as the day wore on, they would start giving me amazing intros in meetings. Stone-faced staffers—already affected by the details of what the responders had witnessed down at Ground Zero, moved by the fact that they continued to come back and do the work and took pride in that work despite facing terrible illness—would think the meeting was wrapping up. Then this group of heroes would turn to me and tell the staffer that I wasn't one of their daughters.

It went like this.

"There were kids down there with us too, you know. You should hear what they went through. We have one with us today."

At this point, the staffer, having already depleted their well of "sad" and "concerned" facial expressions, would sigh. A glimmer of exasperation would flash across their eyes, but, taking their cues from the men seated around them, they'd take a breath, settle in, and listen.

Once you've seen a group of men reduced to tears by their memories of a tragic event, the last thing you want to hear is that kids were there with them. The strategy was impactful.

The FealGood guys made sure I got noticed in every office, every time, even when I blended in with the staffers. The guys also seemed to enjoy my presence between meetings, and the feeling was mutual as we cracked jokes and got lost in the tunnels that connect the Capitol. They insisted I remember to eat lunch, brought me beverages if they thought I wasn't drinking enough water, and patiently waited for me outside the ladies' room all of the six hundred times I had to pee. Our rapport broke up some of the oppressive solemnity. Lobbying with them felt impactful, but it was also fun.

Among the hardworking team of survivor advocates who, like me, rarely got seen in the coverage of the issue, most of us worked double duty like this on some level, lobbying members of Congress from elsewhere in the nation, but also lobbying our own members of Congress and the other advocates. We had to find the openings where we could.

I'm still often ignored or mistaken for a staffer. The number of times a politician has shaken every hand in the room but mine is staggering. It happens with members on both sides of the aisle and of every gender. By 2019, however, I saw the fruits of my labor. On one lobbying day I snuck into a hallway meeting unnoticed and heard a team of responders, most of whom I didn't know, start the student story. My story. They'd heard it from somebody else on their team, which means that many of those responders, guys who were with us kids on and after 9/11, continued to do lifesaving work for us by telling our story even when we weren't there to ask them to.

AT A PRESS CONFERENCE following the successful Senate vote in 2010, a couple of kind, nine-hundred-foot-tall responders pushed me to the front of the crowd so I could watch the speakers and try to be seen in the wide shots. It was hard to get a spot with so many people standing behind the tiny podium, but as I stood up there with their kids, most of whom also towered over me, I heard a very different Senate story than the one we'd been hearing in the late negotiations. It was in front of cameras that I learned that the Zadroga Act, which had been kicking around in some form for years with no success, had largely passed because of Senator Gillibrand, the newly appointed freshman senator from New York. From many senators' snide comments, I pieced together that she was among the most tenacious people any of them had ever encountered. Speaker after speaker described being accosted by her at every waking moment, eventually dreading encounters with her and her staff because they were so persistent on this issue. Senate Majority Leader Harry Reid, who seemed older and frailer in person, described being asked by the beaten-down members of his caucus to bring the bill to a vote so they could get Gillibrand off their backs. One GOP senator, in comments that day, described her as "relentless."[204]

The Senate likes to think of itself as a staid, decorum-obsessed place where everybody is cordial, but it is also a boys' club where female senators get treated the way I often get treated by Senate staffers—like they aren't in the room or maybe work for a man in the room. Senator Gillibrand did not, it seems, go into the Senate with plans to be invited to dinner parties. She went in there to make things happen, knowing that the regular mechanisms of power were probably not going to be accessible to her. For every complaint I've heard on the Hill (in the last decade I've heard many) that she isn't playing by the rules, that her staff doesn't "get" how things get done in the Senate, that she isn't going to be very effective with *that* attitude, I've seen results from her office in the form of real legislation. During the same session she ushered through the Zadroga Act, her first session, I might add, she also played a critical role in the repeal of "Don't Ask, Don't Tell."[205] She's been a ferocious defender of women, even when it's been to her political detriment, calling out men for their sexual misconduct since long before #metoo.[206] As *The New York Times* reported back in 2017,

> Ms. Gillibrand has earned a reputation for aggressively pursuing
> Republican colleagues to sign onto her efforts, from changing
> procedures for reporting sexual assault in the military to rolling out a
> host of Republican co-sponsors this week for a bill to overhaul sexual
> harassment procedures in Congress.[207]

I will never shake the feeling of respect I had for this similarly petite, young-looking woman who hassled and shamed these powerful, self-important men into getting us help. Women have to strategize in unusual ways to get stuff done in male-dominated environments. It's not fair, but it's life. While I was busy lobbying other lobbyists in order to get my story heard, she and her mostly female staff were lobbying colleagues to lobby other colleagues too. It wasn't a miracle that made it happen in either case—it was persistence. We found the openings.

The night the bill finally passed in the Senate she brought us pizza for the bus ride home, and we returned, exhausted, to that dark Midtown corner, where my mother stood in the snow waiting.

CHAPTER 9

THE TOOTH FAIRY
ANGEL OF DEATH

President Obama signed the Zadroga Act into law in January 2011.[208] That year also marked the tenth anniversary of the attacks, and the city and nation were steeped in a giddy commemorative excitement. Americans were encouraged to #NeverForget and buy trinkets and collectible plates brandished with the silhouette of the Twin Towers. The Bush years were over, but America had not shaken its love of solemn 9/11 tributes and wonder-filled speeches about our inspiring national unity. It was, of course, a national unity I didn't quite relate to. New Yorkers were, on some level, the sacrifice other Americans made so they could experience that unity.

For me, rolling unity-free, the year was a little tougher. As those of us on the advocacy side sat with our recent triumph, our excitement evolved into a dawning disappointment that ten years of work had gone into generating only five years of help. It seemed impossible—it had already been an incredibly long haul, comprising my entire adult life up until that point. 9/11's consequences seemed intent on forever reappearing in a loop, never quite resolved.

The press surrounding both the signing of the Zadroga Act and the fervor surrounding the anniversary were good for our outreach efforts for the newly established World Trade Center Health Program, so we did our best to get the information to new people. Because cancers were not yet covered, the outreach was a delicate balancing act. We looked for survivors with asthma, GERD, and PTSD but could offer nothing to people coming forward with serious, fatal illnesses. By the time cancers were added to the list of covered conditions in late 2012, I'd already had to tell a handful of classmates, all suffering the disruption of getting a cancer in their twenties, that their treatment wouldn't be covered, even with the Zadroga Act's passage. I felt a little like a tooth fairy who had a side gig as the angel of death—I could offer a quarter for a tooth but nothing for a life.

I decided to return to New York for the tenth anniversary of September 11 instead of spending it in California, where I was frequently subject to melodramatic 9/11 accounts from people who had no idea about my personal stake in the events. Often they were dismissive or angry when they found out about my advocacy work. There was a sense that advocating for the surviving 9/11 community was somehow disrespectful to those who had been killed in the attacks. New Yorkers had dispensed with that notion, but elsewhere I was frequently met with comments like, "But you weren't a responder" or "It couldn't have been that bad" or "But other people lost people that day."

In the Stuyvesant community, many of us avoided delving into 9/11 as a topic for years. I still am not clear on the details of how some of my closest friends evacuated or what they were feeling when we returned on that weirdly chaotic October day. I have no idea where my best friend spent that terrifying night. We supported each other in different ways, treating our friends with patience as they jumped at loud noises or had oddly extreme reactions to smells and crowds and the sight of airplanes flying overhead, making a silent promise that we wouldn't talk about our fears about violence and the future if we couldn't deal with facing them, or sometimes even expressing a willingness to be defiantly unafraid together in a crowd as other Americans worried about the looming threat of new terrorist attacks. We never spoke of that day, however. Even now I would rather tell Congress about my evacuation than somebody for whom the story has personal resonance. One of the struggles of doing outreach work on this issue has always been balancing the desire to never speak of 9/11 again with the need to address its consequences.

Nevertheless, I was pleased, though surprised, when I was contacted by a group of Stuyvesant alumni interested in putting on an event for the anniversary. Not only would it save all of us from having to attend memorials or even work drinks that evening with people who didn't "get it," but it would give me a chance to see how my efforts to animate the health care discussion were being received by other alumni. By this point StuyHealth was mostly an email list through which I sent out information and calls to action. I hoped it was not becoming a nagging reminder to the student body to feel traumatized.

The event's organizing committee was composed of the usual suspects—former student government types and people active in the alumni association. In discussing where to hold it we immediately encountered an unsurprising obstacle: Stanley Teitel, the law-and-order-loving Stuyvesant principal who'd defended our return back in 2001 and had stayed consistent on the matter since. Our alumni group approached him about using the school's theater and, after a frustrating back and forth during which he rejected our request, then tried to pass the buck to another city entity, he finally told us that he simply couldn't understand why alumni would want to memorialize the day together.[209] "Why would [students] want to relive that day?" he told Gothamist during the back-and-forth. "I certainly don't want to relive that day. . . . And they just happened to be [at the school on 9/11]—why do they want to be here?"[210] A confounding response.

We had some support on the inside, luckily. Several teachers and ex-teachers also wanted to participate, and they helped us find another route, going over his head to apply pressure to the Battery Park City Authority, which controlled use of the school's facilities after hours. Teitel abided by their ultimate decision to let us use the space, though I was struck by how every teacher, both young and old, was united in their frustration with him—a frustration not only with how the school was being run in 2011 but with how insensitive his administration had been about this difficult date and every anniversary since 2001. It was their trauma too, and just as he had the power to set policy for us students, he'd had this power over them as well.

Unlike the teachers, some of the organizing committee's alumni were relatively shocked by Teitel's attempts to throw up obstacles. I wasn't. He did the same thing every time he was approached with a 9/11-related ask. That ten-year anniversary capped many years of my own attempts to reach out to his office, attempts that almost always fell on deaf ears. His administration wouldn't cooperate with our efforts to alert the student body about the 9/11 health risks or the city, state, or federal services available. Their suspicion of us bled into our relationship with the alumni association, which was run by older alumni who didn't understand the scale of the 9/11 problem and weren't very interested in hearing about it because it wasn't going to help them raise money. We'd made repeated attempts to get notices put in the alumni newsletter, to have emails go out to the affected class years about the health services, and had worked with other outreach groups to educate his office about the situation. I was the only 9/11 health advocate who ever got an actual meeting with him, but it was a bit of a bust.

Our meeting took place in mid-2006, just as StuyHealth was getting off the ground. We met in his first-floor office—a space I'd never spent much time in as a student. It was a huge room with a large desk, a plush couch, and trophies everywhere. I wasn't sure what to call him—I wanted to be treated like an adult but didn't want to be disrespectful—so I tried not to use his name at all as I weakly shook his hand. I sat uncomfortably on a couch so large my feet barely reached the ground. I told him we could use his help getting word out to alumni about the risks we'd faced.

"We want to contact every student from the era but don't have access to email lists, to rosters of the student body from that time, to any students who don't live in the area and aren't on social media."

He was listening but resistant. "We can't just give that information out."

I wasn't asking for something political. It wasn't a personal favor. I was asking for a PSA. I wanted the school to send out a mass email, letting everybody know to check our website or opt in for more information. He, oddly, reacted as if I was requesting special treatment and told me that they couldn't allow alumni to send emails to the entire student body about just anything.

When I responded that the health risks were directly related to something that happened to us in school, he answered that they couldn't have done anything differently at the time.

I held my tongue.

Finally, he asked, "How many students are sick?" Always that question. Even from the people standing in the way of our getting the answer. But we couldn't find out without help contacting former students.

He eventually told me to talk to the Parents' Association, and when I responded that we were already working with them, he said that I should talk to a doctor and ask them to start a research project.

"Does that preclude us from sending out an email?" I asked him.

He said he'd think about it. He didn't want to alarm people.

In retrospect, I can see that Teitel was also a victim of the situation in his own way. He was a guy who respected authority, even when it was to his own detriment, and since he liked to follow orders, he'd followed them on 9/11. On that day and the days that followed, however, the orders were coming from people who didn't have enough information to make the appropriate calls. Unfortunately, he lacked the leadership skills to stand up for himself or for those of us in his care. Still, while it's petty to say, it was satisfying, given all I'd faced because of him, to get to hold our commemorative event in his house while he was still in charge. (He, of course, made sure to be away from the premises.)

TEITEL, IT TURNED OUT, was the only person who couldn't put together why we'd want to hold the event at Stuyvesant. A Facebook group that was set up to publicize the plan quickly racked up twelve hundred members. Considering how many alumni were no longer living in New York, the turnout on the day was equally impressive.

The event was organized haphazardly with a speaker's sign-up sheet that anybody could add their name to. We weren't really sure how it would go—whether a lot of people would want to speak or whether we'd all sit in an awkward silence. I made an announcement at the beginning about StuyHealth and manned a table in the back with some hastily thrown-to-gether palm cards and an email sign-up sheet. I had never really needed to put together materials—most of my work was online—so I slapped a terri-ble logo I'd created to make official letterhead for a letter to Congress onto a Microsoft Word document about the WTC Health Program and sent it to print overnight at Kinko's. I also brought some swag from the World Trade Center Environmental Health Center run by Health & Hospitals Corporation—pens with tiny flashlights on them and tote bags. I put them next to the cards (which the staff at Kinko's had bizarrely chosen to print on glossy photo paper) to fill out the display and did my best to aggressively force the swag onto passersby. Most of the pens came home with me that night. I've been finding the remnants of that event around my house for years. The tiny flashlights have been useful during blackouts.

Swag woes aside, the event was a huge success. We did not wind up sitting in silence and staring at our feet. People were, it seemed, ready to talk, at least to a sympathetic audience of their 9/11 peers. I was struck by how many of the speakers said that they'd never spoken about their 9/11 experience with anybody before. One speaker acknowledged that every-body has a different way of processing that day and that their method has been avoidance. Another conceded that his best friend couldn't attend the event because he gets emotional when he talks about 9/11. A lowerclass-man from the era recounted his first moments after being told a plane had hit the World Trade Center, during which he'd pictured a rickety, small, red, single-engine propeller airplane crashing into the buildings like a toy.

"I could not fathom a situation in which someone would purposely fly the plane into a building. It didn't exist to me. I couldn't accept that serious reality, so I only went to the ludicrous joke. And I remember making that joke in my classroom and I remember a girl crying to my right because her sister was in that building and she was worried for her safety and we had absolutely no information. And I remember for years feeling incredibly guilty because the way I coped made the way she coped that much worse."

There were a few awkward moments. At one point a 9/11-era parent— the only one I saw in attendance—got up, obviously still grappling with his role in our quick return. After talking about the dissention within the PA and how our presence downtown during the cleanup had imperiled our health, he boldly said, "Were there villains? Absolutely there were villains. It would be untrue to say that there were no bona fide villains. But what's important is to find forgiveness." As if the decision to bestow forgiveness didn't belong to us, the ones living with the aftermath. As if it was something we should be forced to do. And whose forgiveness was he asking for? His own?

By far the most memorable speech that day was made by Pam Council, a junior on 9/11. She spoke about the broken escalator phenomenon. The phenomenon involves the sensation of imbalance that occurs when someone walks onto a broken escalator. Even though they are aware that it is broken, they still instinctively speed up when they step on, losing balance as they awkwardly try to walk on the stationary stairs with the forward-tilting posture of an escalator rider. She used the premise as a metaphor for our adaptability, asserting that because of our experiences around September 11 and also because of our many days spent traversing the school building's many actual broken escalators, Stuy students were resilient, able to shift and adapt to any situation. While some people might get tripped up by a broken escalator, we were able to keep it moving. She closed saying, of the metaphor, "If one person gets it and is with me on it, then I've done my job." Everybody got it.

Much to my relief, plenty of people also came up to me to thank me for my work or discuss what StuyHealth was doing. I was pleased to learn that I wasn't single-handedly ruining lives by sending out emails about health concerns and lobbying days. Even in our school-wide avoidance, people had been slowly learning the disquieting facts about the WTC cleanup, were scared about the future, and were glad somebody (and, let's be honest, somebody else) was bringing it up. I thought back to the spring of 2007, those days when I thought I'd walk away from it all. I was glad I hadn't.

AS THE FEDERAL HEALTH services expanded, our outreach and education obligations did as well. There was a lot to keep up with in late 2011 and early 2012, adding to what was already a confusing time for me personally. My father got a job teaching at a university in Lebanon, and my parents moved to Beirut very suddenly in the fall of 2011, subletting my New York crash pad to strangers. I joined them in Beirut at the end of the year, staying into late January 2012, doing my best to eke out a vacation while I could. They had an apartment on the top floor of a dorm building in a neighborhood called Hamra, a cute commercial hilltop squeezed between two large American universities. My mother was retired and didn't know anybody, so we spent the days walking for miles along the Mediterranean, enjoying the warm breeze and sunshine, and watching kids play in the splashes of surf that would spray the boardwalk on windy days. Periodically we'd call a taxi, usually the same one driven by a jovial man we spoke to in broken French, and go to some far-flung part of town to explore. We ate pastries in the French Quarter and bought new clothes at the mall that sat atop the ancient Souk. We celebrated Orthodox and regular Christmas in their small kitchen, listening to a mix of weird pop Christmas carols playing on a loop from a store downstairs, sometimes competing with the call to prayer.

I returned to Los Angeles by way of New York, staying with friends and family in Brooklyn and Queens. I didn't see the city for another six months.

For a while, in the flux created by my parents' move, I was without access to asthma care. I had been grandfathered into the federal WTC Health Program because I was a patient at the Bellevue clinic already, but there wasn't yet care available outside of New York City, and I was temporarily without a place to call home there. I passed time in LA trying to learn about the new application process so I could assist other people. Things were often confusing, since, as is the case with most government programs, there were always new and sometimes complicated layers of jargon and bureaucracy to wade through, documentation obstacles to face. To apply for care, patients had to provide proof of presence. While students could send school transcripts, kids who didn't attend school downtown ran into obstacles when it came to furnishing adequate legal documentation to prove their presence. Could you prove your whereabouts as a toddler? Especially now, decades later, when it might mean tracking down a caregiver's decades-old utility bills or long-forgotten leases. Or seeking the help of parents who might be estranged or deceased. It is one of the most distressing and difficult-to-troubleshoot issues that some survivors face.

As the procedures for getting health services evolved, having the 9/11 side gig became more difficult for less geography-related reasons as well. At the beginning of 2012, for the first time, I took a full-time, noncontingent, could-just-go-on-forever-and-ever job in LA. The job was in entertainment but had traditional job-like qualities such as requiring me to go into an office (a cubicle!), wear the dreaded business casual attire, and sit at a bulky desktop PC with a tendency to crash randomly while running an old version of MS Windows. Up until that point I'd been freelancing—my nascent writing career was launched by that 2008 *Guardian* essay on 9/11—but it was hard to find consistent work in that or any other field. I had been bouncing around a lot and not finding anywhere to land.

I would have, frankly, happily continued to do that, but my health insurance situation forced my hand. It's a common story that only exists in America. A couple of years prior, my insurance rates had spiked and I'd tried to switch insurers. Because of my 9/11-related issues—chronic but not wholly uncommon issues like asthma and GERD—I'd been rejected by every insurance provider in California. Every. Single. One.

By the end of 2011, because of these rejections, I was being forced to pay huge sums to my insurer, Anthem Blue Shield, to stay on my original health plan. They were empowered to raise my premiums to any amount, and I had no recourse because I could not get insurance elsewhere. For somebody with chronic health needs, this was incredibly distressing. It put my access to basic care and the World Trade Center Health Program, which requires care for survivors to be first run through a primary insurer, at risk. In that era, a lot of people facing this same set of concerns were forced to go without insurance. Others were forced to stay at exploitative jobs in order to keep the employer-provided insurance they had. My choice was pretty clear. I could use up all my savings paying off Anthem for increasingly bad coverage or I could find a job that offered insurance, even if it wasn't a good fit. It took a while, but in early 2012, I found one. It was poorly paid, dead-end, at a desk located in a cubicle *inside a server closet* at a major Hollywood talent agency, but I had no real choice.

To keep myself sane, I viewed the job as essentially another freelance gig that was going to carry me into the year where the Affordable Care Act would nullify the laws allowing companies to reject people with preexisting conditions.[211] I knew that if I gave up my Anthem plan I would need to stay in the new job for well over a year or risk having no access to insurance. When a more temporary job that I really did want came up the next month, I had to turn it down. When it turned out the boss at the job with benefits was abusive and erratic, I had to stay. Then, as 2012 continued, I realized a few other things had been wrong with my strategy. For one, care never became particularly affordable to me under the ACA. Premiums remained hundreds of dollars a month, in some places even outstripping costs under the old system.[212] The subsidies offered by the ACA were minimal and insufficient, especially in high cost-of-living areas like Los Angeles.[213] The scope of coverage was certainly better, and starting in 2014 somebody like me could finally buy insurance, but given the minimal federal assistance, high out-of-pocket costs on most of the plans, and constant attempts by politicians to strip out protections, the system wasn't meaningfully stable or affordable for people in my situation.

Then, the rest of my exit strategy fell apart. A TV showrunner whom I'd been working with on and off and had promised would take me with him onto his next show died under tragic circumstances. I found myself without anywhere to go, depressed and stuck. I still wanted to write, still wanted to rejoin the creative class, but I was coming home brain dead, devoting what little energy I had to 9/11 outreach work, and was too crushed to care about the future. I stayed for years longer than expected and did my best to stay abreast of the conversation in New York, living a bizarre double life in health advocacy that nobody knew about at my "real" job.

There was one bright spot in that period, though. In October 2012, the Nationwide Provider Network finally launched.[214] Inside the 9/11 advocacy community not much was known about when this national component of the WTC Health Program would open its doors and how it would function, but those of us outside of New York had been waiting for it with bated breath. I became one of its earliest survivor patients and spent a lot of time on the phone with advocates and the program managers trying to troubleshoot some initial issues.

I'd never been a part of a program launch and had never been asked to give feedback about the performance of a newly developed bureaucracy, and being the only young person in that phone tree was a bizarre experience. Many of the early National Program issues did not arise because the people involved in the network were intentionally creating these difficulties, but because the program was set up with responders, not younger people, in mind.

The Nationwide Provider Network is a part of the World Trade Center Health Program, but it isn't managed by the government directly. It's managed by a company in Wisconsin that contracts with a private insurer's medical network to find doctors, meaning it has two layers of additional corporate bureaucracy beyond the usual government bureaucratic fare. The company, LHI, mostly manages social security and veteran's benefits, and their work with the 9/11 community is overseen by a government office based in Atlanta.

Atlanta. Wisconsin. From what I could tell, the first major program-level problem was just that there weren't many New Yorkers involved. It's not because I think we're so special (fine, we are) but because when you're creating a resource that will be serving a huge population of New Yorkers and ex–New Yorkers, it's helpful to know what makes them tick. It reminded me a little of the NYC Department of Health's 9/11 Health Registry survey and my awkward chat with that call center in the Deep South.

The program launch had some immediate issues. LHI had no online component, so there was no way to get appointment information without making a phone call. That meant that when the program had information to share, they would do so by leaving a cryptic phone message that required making a return call or by sending a signature-required FedEx package with documents. Generally, return calls led to a voicemail box, and then their return call for your return call, if you got one, would take place at the weirdest possible time because LHI wasn't in the same time zone as most of its World Trade Center patients. The FedExed documents system was even more mystifying. Who was going to be home to sign for all of those mailings? How could there be no electronic way to transmit names and addresses for doctor's appointments? What did I not understand about federal law that required daily FedExing? And who was paying for all of that rush mailing?

The program was also shocked when I raised the issue of the LHI phone greetings, which involved their incredibly cheerful staff repeating an outrageous amount of introductory information. As a young adult who already hated being on the phone, I'd find myself sitting in silence for five minutes before getting a chance to speak as the staff rattled off the name of the program (which in its shortest form was still "The World Trade Center Health Program Nationwide Provider Network") and other information, only to then launch into a series of polite small-talk-style questions before finally getting to the point.

The differing role small talk plays in certain American contexts was one of the major cultural distinctions I had noticed after moving to California. I had some insight into the small-talk thing from my Iowan-raised best friend in LA. When he calls or texts me, he often pesters (though he might say "engages") me with a long series of polite questions before telling me his specific reason for getting in touch. The more mundane the information he's trying to share, the worse the small talk is and the more annoyed I get because it feels like he is deliberately wasting my time. I spent years wondering why he was doing this until one day I watched his incredibly nice dad butter up a grocery store employee for twenty minutes just to ask where the orange juice was. That's when it occurred to me that my friend wasn't trying to be cagey, he was actually trying to be polite. In some areas of the country, you can't just ask people something without indicating that you care about how they are. To a New Yorker, this is more likely perceived as wasting the person's time—the height of local imprudence.

When I started getting calls from StuyHealth members complaining to me that they couldn't navigate the LHI phone tree, I began suspecting that it had something to do with this issue. I was on those calls too, after all, and I would find my patience tested the same way. A subtle difference in regional etiquette was hampering our calls to LHI and our ability to interact with the WTC Health Program. As silly and harmless as this misunderstanding would be in real life, it's incredibly enraging when unnecessary small talk happens on a long, boring call that is also related to an upsetting major trauma. I argued vehemently that the LHI staffers had to start talking faster and getting to the point faster. Everybody treated me like I was being melodramatic. Many told me variations on, "There are things you can change and things you can't," as if the phone greeting was the one program tradition that, once enacted, could never be changed. Some projected my comment onto their larger Georgia/Wisconsin disdain for New Yorkers, implying that they were offended that an annoying New Yorker was trying to tell them how to talk when everybody knows New Yorkers are rude anyway. Still, those silly notes made a huge difference in how the program was experienced by those of us it was trying to serve. Sometimes being a good advocate just means agreeing to be embarrassed.

Awkward demands aside, I took this role of giving what I dubbed my "bureaucracy notes" very seriously. The Nationwide Provider Network was conceived of as a service mostly for responders, but young people were the survivor group with the biggest stake in it. We were all at the precipice of a major life change when 9/11 happened. Every year, thousands of students went away to college, then scattered with the wind as life and New York City's outrageous rents conspired to keep us away. Many of us were seeing doctors in other states that had no knowledge of 9/11's environmental consequences and desperately needed access to this program to get any quality of care for our conditions. This was especially true on the mental health front—often mental health care isn't meaningfully covered by insurance, even in the post-ACA era,[215] but it's something a lot of 9/11 survivors and, in fact, survivors of most traumas, desperately need.[216]

IN A VICTORY FOR Amit and the many classmates who had come forward with cancers since, 2012 was also the year that the first cancers were added to the program's list of covered conditions. Because cancers took so long to make the list and because the serious nature of having cancer is such that you don't want to take a wild risk with your care, people often didn't want or think to go to the program for their treatment—which meant most of them were asking me about the Victim Compensation Fund instead. It's funny to say now, given that I've devoted over a year of my life to educating Congress about the VCF, a major component of the Zadroga Act, but at the time I didn't understand the program. I didn't know who qualified or on what grounds. A lot of us seemed to be in the dark about that. One former classmate was a lawyer who seemed to vaguely understand the nuts and bolts and offered to assist StuyHealth members with the process, so, when I got questions, I passed them on to him, directing sick classmates to an alum in Florida they barely knew. They'd call him armed with only the information that he was a cancer survivor because, frankly, that was also all I could tell them.

Confusion about the VCF was common in the broader survivor community as well, but even so, crazed warnings would periodically be passed around our email lists reminding us that we had to "register" before 2013 so we didn't "lose our spot in line." I didn't know what that meant, though I shared the warnings just the same and "registered" myself, not really knowing why. I eventually knew to direct cancer survivors to look into the program but wasn't sure what to say beyond "you might want to find a lawyer." Nobody mentioned that nonfatal chronic conditions might be compensable. The burden of proof on the patient sounded insurmountable, and the legalese on the VCF's website was intimidating.

I also admit I also didn't ask for clarification. I was used to hearing that an arbitrary deadline might stop us from getting some service or another—that's what happens when a crisis response is put together piecemeal. We'd already faced a lot of random deadlines, regulations, and limitations as 9/11 survivors. I was, for example, used to hearing from classmates that they wanted to participate in research but couldn't get into the WTC Health Registry because it had been closed since 2006, long before they even were aware of the discussion about health concerns and exposure. In that context, the VCF deadline in 2013 felt like yet another opportunity that we kids would miss out on because we weren't sick enough or aware enough fast enough. Like there was a downpour coming but all the doors and windows were closing before we could get inside.

CHAPTER 10

NEVER ENOUGH

I left my "real job" job in May 2015 and began working on a short-run TV series. It was a desperate, last-minute bid to get out of my windowless basement office and spend the summer around people. Any people. The new gig was on the set of a multi-cam sitcom, the kind with a live audience and snacks everywhere and paid-for lunches brought in from a new restaurant every day. I worked in a roach-infested trailer on the Fox Lot that smelled, and somehow also looked, damp, but the supply of sugary cereals was bottomless, and once a week I'd walk to the studio a few buildings down to find some previously unremarkable empty corner transformed into a high school basketball court or an apartment or a hospital. I would marvel at how all of that change had been accomplished overnight. Television production is a never-ending cycle of fresh starts.

My new office was nothing glamorous—it was basically a hallway that I shared with two recent college graduates—but I basked in the novelty of having a small, square window twenty feet from my desk with a view of the outdoors or, more accurately, an open-air loading dock for the studio lighting warehouse. The recent grads passed long days asking me about the wisdom I'd accrued at my advanced age (that age being thirty years old). I explained health insurance. Laid out the costs that accompany car ownership. Discovered I was the only person in the hallway whose groceries were coming out of my meager paycheck, not a parent's bank account. Sometimes I felt arrested in time, forced to relive the confusion of my early twenties for their benefit, but those drawbacks were unimportant. I was burned out from the business-casual windowless closet I'd spent the last three and a half years in and happy the new job was short-term. A fresh start, but with a quick expiration date. Just like the high school basketball court set.

The new gig was mercifully casual. My first act upon walking out of the agency job for the last time had been to push my rigidly formal office wear to the back of my closet. A suit-wearer no more! I planned to never lay eyes on any of those slacks and button-downs again, spending my last weekend of freedom researching what jeans people were wearing these days and quickly relaxing into a new sweatshirt and sneakers existence. I bought new shoes to look the part, and after years of blistery ballet flats and heels, they seemed like the most comfortable things I had ever slipped onto my feet.

It was, unfortunately, only a couple of weeks into my newly window-filled life that I found myself hesitantly digging slacks out of my closet again. I carefully tiptoed up to my brand-new boss's desk in the show's production office and asked if I could have a few days off to go to New York and participate in a Federal Advisory Committee meeting related to 9/11 health concerns. She looked at me like I had three heads. "You have a very interesting life, Lila" was all she mustered up in response.

I'D WAITED SO LONG for this meeting that it seemed unlikely to ever happen. I had been nominated to serve on the World Trade Center Scientific and Technical Advisory Committee, STAC for short, back in 2013. It's a body that advises the head of the WTC Health Program, and though we'd done one teleconference in early 2014, it was not until January 2015 that we finally got a date for our first in-person summit, June 4. I'd neglected to mention it when I interviewed for the new job, not wanting to raise questions about what somebody with my credentials was doing interviewing for an assistant position in television. A month later, when somebody finally asked that exact question, I replied that I didn't want to remember the worst day of my life for a living. She didn't make eye contact with me for a week. People are so weird about 9/11.

The STAC meeting felt like a completely different life. The other members were primarily doctors with specialties related to environmental or occupational health. A few community representatives and responders were thrown in for good measure. I was the first young survivor appointed, though as the appointment dragged on without so much as a peep from the committee staff, I started to wonder if I'd been booted over a missing qualification. Maybe it was like the presidency where you had to be at least thirty-five years old? Just before the June meeting, information suddenly started coming fast and furious, and the whole thing became very exciting. I was flown, like a real professional, to the meeting. In my life then, just being put on a real airplane, even if it was in a middle seat in the back row, seemed like an outrageous extravagance. Then there were the nameplates, professionally printed on thick plastic placards, awaiting each participant at a long, U-shaped table facing a podium and audience seating. They lent a feeling of weight to the assignment.

The June meeting was a day and a half long and held at the Jacob K. Javits Federal Building in Lower Manhattan, confusingly close in name (and not in location) to the Jacob K. Javits Convention Center in Midtown. It was a small miracle that I even wound up in the right place. Getting into the building involved a lot of frustrating security procedures and rules. The removing of shoes and belts. A request for printed-out paperwork. Appropriate ID. An argument with a humorless guard since the paperwork they wanted was not the paperwork we had.

Once we were inside, the federal government did its best to keep the minor inconvenience level high. To avoid ethical issues, they don't allow anybody to provide food or beverages at the meetings, not even water bottles, so snacks had to be brought or purchased on premises. Assuming you'd purchased your own, you would be asked to leave all food items at the door. Only water was allowed in the meeting room itself. The snacks and lunch were stored in an unrefrigerated lounge where you couldn't actually reach them.

STAC meetings, as it turned out, are also quite long. In my seven years on the committee, most lasted only one day, slightly shorter than that first meeting, but all still involved three to four presentations on very technical research topics as well as occasional long-winded PowerPoint presentations, which tend to be, let's be honest, boring no matter the subject. (One of the saving graces of working in Hollywood is that, even while being underpaid and exploited, overworked and yelled at, nobody has ever forced me to watch a PowerPoint heavily featuring empty jargon and arrows that serve no purpose.)

But the nameplates. They were so solid and glossy. They were everything.

When I was a child, my father made industrial films and would often be flown to medical conventions at fancy resorts, sometimes taking us along to enjoy the free accommodations. I remember tiptoeing by those conference rooms with my mother on our way to the pool, catching glimpses of thousands of doctors watching more important doctors address them from behind large nameplates at tables on the stage, like a university lecture hall on steroids. The nameplates made me feel like I was at the head of one of those tables.

Being on STAC and sitting in that room with those doctors and researchers was sometimes intimidating, but it was incredibly helpful to my work. There is an aspect to being an advocate in the long term that you don't think about in the beginning, when being effective is largely about having a sense of justice and a knack for theater. Over time the work becomes more formalized and institutionalized. At some point you have to follow through on your demands and oversee the programs those demands create. That part of the process often requires advocates to develop at least a working understanding of some subject areas that other people go to school for years to learn about. Advocating for yourself to scientists and doctors is different from advocating to politicians. What begin as fiery speeches on the steps of the Capitol can evolve into carefully meted questions involving "comorbidity," or comments in accord with a point about IRB (institutional review board) protocol. (Also it always, always involves learning new acronyms.)

I'd joined STAC as a lay expert in health care policy because I'd had to become one to survive my twenties, but the world of research was a different animal. Research, like health policy, is inherently political since *who* we research and *why* are often based on whom we value as a society and why.[217] The language around medical research, however, sounds significantly more impartial. Understanding how politics are couched in the language of scientific merit requires some experience, and serving on STAC helped me develop that experience. Eventually I morphed into the kind of person that can hold an entire conversation about gender imbalances in research and how to choose representative cohorts. That person gets taken much more seriously in meetings than the twenty-five-year-old activist she replaced.

A COUPLE OF DAYS after the STAC meeting I returned to California. The new job carried on well past August, stretching month by month without an end date but also without any promises that it would continue. The stand-up comedian I had been assisting on the show hired me directly and kept me on from home after the first season ended to keep track of his schedule. I was happier with the set-up than I expected—I hated being an assistant, but I liked being home and getting to flit from TV to 9/11 to shopping at Target whenever I wanted.

Something about the job was also a good antidote to the depressing health news I receive on a regular basis from classmates, other advocates, and my New York community in general. Comedians are mostly depressed—a lot of comedy is derived from personal pain—but the brief moments of levity that accompany working in the general airspace of comedy were helpful to me. My boss's approach to comedy—his shtick involved making boldly impassive remarks about controversial topics and traumatic events—was a helpful break from the enforced solemnity of my 9/11 life. Back during that first TV season together, as we got to know each other, I'd let him ask me about my 9/11 experience in detail. I had the sense that he wanted to mine my story for material, but I'd agreed out of curiosity. He set aside a date for our conversation and made it oddly official, waving people out of the room when they stopped by like we were in an important meeting. The only other person who joined us was his writing partner, and the two of them goaded me into performing my 9/11 story like a stand-up set. They leaned in to what was most disturbing about the account, unselfconsciously asking for clarifications about what a falling body looks like, what an asthmatic run looks like, what a burning building smells like. Their tone was light. #NeverForget was not a solemn refrain; it was the joke.

The conversation, in its retelling, sounds insensitive and cruel, but how it actually felt was cathartic. They didn't treat the story with kid gloves, but it meant I didn't have to either. I was honest about how much of my work was being fueled by anger. How the plaintive search for justice act was sometimes just for the cameras, masking a growing, morphing fury, not just at a system that didn't acknowledge the costs they'd imposed on us but at a system that didn't treat us as valuable victims even when they knew the costs. I unleashed a monologue that wasn't fit for television news. I was, briefly, a bad team player. A bad politician. They didn't bat an eye, just dug in further. My boss loved it, perhaps for the wrong reasons, but I felt freed by that experience. We had a pretty good working relationship after that.

When word got around the office that I'd been forced to have that 9/11 conversation, it was clear that I was meant to act put-upon. The sad, concerned looks I got for the rest of the week made that known. (It was Hollywood, so of course nobody said anything to the boss.) I never told anybody outside the office about that day, fearing they'd develop that sad look too. Oddly, however, it was the conversation that, to me, finally validated my move to LA. Being solemn is exhausting. You need a way to exist that allows you to make an honest joke about your traumatic past. You need an audience that will allow for an impactful tragedy in your life to also be the punch line of a joke and won't bat an eye when the punch line sounds harsher than you intended.

I agreed to stay on in the assistant job, but I mentioned a caveat up front. I had to take time off to be in New York for the 9/11 anniversary. It was a big year. In early September I started to get information about the lobbying efforts being planned around the anniversary's commemorative activities because, just like that, our five years were already up. The Zadroga Act was set to expire at the end of the year. Caught in the haze of my new life in television three thousand miles away from the action, I'd been out of the loop, but I felt a pull to jump back in.

Though Rep. Carolyn Maloney and Sen. Kirsten Gillibrand's expansively named James Zadroga 9/11 Health and Compensation Reauthorization Act of 2015, which aimed to permanently extend the 2010 act, had been introduced in both chambers on April 14, 2015,[218] September was our opportunity to capitalize on the anniversary fervor and draw public attention to the cause. Events were being planned in DC on September 16, and according to other advocates, the date was going to be a big deal in the media because of a secret celebrity guest. Jon Stewart, after playing a vital role in the 2010 renewal efforts from the inside of his *Daily Show* studios, had agreed to headline an informational gathering being organized for Senate staffers.[219] With Stewart as the main draw, the attendees would be asked to listen to stories from critically ill responders about the WTC recovery efforts and the experience of getting sick in the aftermath. The hope was that they would accidentally find out how important the Zadroga Act was while trying to see Jon Stewart tell jokes. The coalition organizing the event, spearheaded by a 501(c)(4) run by Rep. Maloney's former chief of staff,[220] needed to make at least a nod to the survivor community, so, much to my surprise, I was invited to speak.

The morning of September 16, I met a team of survivor advocates at Penn Station at 5:00 a.m. NYC Health + Hospitals (at the time known as Health & Hospitals Corporation or HHC), which runs the World Trade Center Environmental Health Center in New York, had gotten us train tickets on the Acela, an outrageous luxury to my half-broke, bus-taking self. Between that and my STAC flights, I was really basking in the glory of a newfound professionalism. It clashed with my identity as the glorified travel agent to a twentysomething stand-up comedian who refused to fly coach, but it was something.

Then we missed the train. Thanks to an incorrect announcement and the fact that it was 5:00 a.m. so nobody in our group was at their sharpest, we boarded, discovered we were erroneously sitting on a train heading to Boston, quickly disembarked just in time to avoid going hours out of our way, but missed our own train in the process. I was forced to sit for an extra hour at Penn Station with the giddy energy of somebody who is just about to meet her icon and the crushing anxiety of somebody who is concerned she might miss her shot.

I had seen Jon in the flesh a couple of times before, but only as an audience member at tapings of *The Daily Show*, which my mother and I would periodically attend on a whim, and during that bizarre weekend in 2010 when I crammed 9/11 lobbying and the Rally to Restore Sanity into a single trip. He was, for me and for most of my generation, larger than life. I was right in the sweet spot of Clinton/Bush-era teens who grew up getting our news from *The Daily Show* and election updates from the "Indecision [insert current year]" segment. Elections had been my sport since childhood, but much of my interest in the seemingly dull machinations of polling and stumping was honed by watching Jon Stewart pick them apart on *The Daily Show*. Even on days where the news was just too depressing, I could always stomach Jon Stewart's take.

On that day in September 2015, my goal was simple and straightforward. I would get a picture. Easy-peasy.

We arrived late, just after the morning press conference, totally flustered, not really sure what the schedule of the day was or how to find somebody who might know. Some staffers had clearly been looking for me, because the instant I set foot on the lawn where the team was dispersing, I was whisked away from my travel mates and sent to one of the Capitol office buildings.

My photo goal, as it turned out, was too simple. I accomplished it within minutes of entering the conference room in which speakers and their family members were awaiting the event's start. I saw Jon Stewart at the end of the table, asked one of the responder advocates to introduce us, and we took the picture. I smiled, thanked him, then ate a granola bar in the corner and beamed to myself while a bunch of responder family members stared at me quizzically, probably trying to figure out whose daughter I was.

The picture was, ultimately, small potatoes. The day morphed from there into what remains, to this day, the most exciting day of my life. Peak, life-changing, remember-on-my-deathbed excitement.

THE STAFFER SEMINAR THAT kicked everything off went well. A large crowd turned up, and Jon gave remarks that towed the line between displaying his amusement at and disappointment in everybody there. The staffers laughed, but there was an uncomfortable tinge to their applause. They'd expected him to be more fun. Less angry. When John Feal, our responder advocate-in-chief, spoke in his usual evocative style, the room began to deflate. He mentioned the many friends he'd lost, ricocheting between shouts and tears. Periodically he directed comments to the crowd. "We rushed in to protect this country and we were proud to. Now it's your turn to protect us."

Next up, a couple of responders told their personal stories of heroism and illness. They were cancer survivors and described, also through tears, the scene they'd responded to on 9/11, the extreme health problems they'd suffered from, their shock at getting their diagnoses. I'm always startled by the graphic detail responders are trained and willing to go into. Taking their cues from John Feal, they allowed their emotions to take charge. Fixing my face with a sad expression and tuning out the sad stories in an attempt to protect a shred of the mental bandwidth I would need to tell my own, I looked on as the crowd of staffers, young and eagerly professional, slowly morphed into a sea of scared teenagers. A massive collection of grief and sadness. Periodically, I noticed impassive glares interspersed among the growing tearful faces. I assumed that they, like me, had tuned out to protect themselves.

I probably didn't look like a 9/11 victim, sitting among these tall men in uniforms and badges. I looked like a fellow staffer. I was very self-conscious about that and a little distracted by the many looks of confusion as I went up to speak. The mic was much too high, and as I lowered it, I made the fatal mistake of noticing my hands. They had nothing to do. Nowhere to be. A surge of adrenaline hit me as I stood at the now head-level mic. Then panic. I had gotten so caught up in the excitement of meeting Jon Stewart that I had not prepared anything to say. I almost forgot how to introduce myself as I sped through my usual spiel, barely stopping to take a breath. Halfway through I caught John Feal's eye and he gestured at me to slow down, so I took a moment to regroup. I told my story but made sure to note everything that made my situation uniquely relatable to the occupants of that room, filled, as it was, with my contemporaries.

"I think I'm the same age as a lot of you. This was what I had to go through just to go to school." I watched their faces slowly drop again. Just as in the lobbying meetings, hearing me on the heels of a series of strong men breaking down in tears made it all seem worse.

I don't remember who made the final pitch. I zoned out after I sat down, still high on the adrenaline. Whoever it was, probably John or Jon, made a final call to action, urging staffers to push their bosses to support our bill. Jon Stewart made a final joke. Then we filed out.

I assumed the responders and Jon would ditch me at this point. That was how those things usually went. The celebrity would be whisked into important meetings while you were sent off to beg unresponsive offices to do things that they had no intention of doing. Sensing that this moment with Jon Stewart was probably a once-in-a-lifetime chance, I resolved to stay with the group until I was specifically asked to stop following them, determined to be the kind of head-in-the-sand, pesky person who refuses to take a hint. My hell-bent persistence wasn't necessary. We quickly formed a little lobbying brigade, Jon Stewart as our entrée into every office, and spent the rest of the day doing drop-in visits and guerilla lobbying around the Capitol.

Being on the Hill with Jon Stewart is a different animal than being on the Hill as a regular person. Doors opened for him with startling ease, and, by extension, they opened for us: the ragtag bunch traveling with him. Early in the day, Jon accosted Sen. Patty Murray of Washington, the Democratic head of the Senate Health, Education, Labor & Pensions Committee, in the hallway. We got a meeting with her (not just her staff—the senator herself) a few hours later. We spoke to a gathering of representatives on the House side as well, which, much to my amazement, was populated not by staffers but by members of Congress themselves, all excited to meet Jon Stewart. We ate lunch together in the congressional cafeteria, just Jon, a couple of responder buddies, and myself, during which I had the chance to casually gab about politics with the man who had taught me how to follow an election.

Some of the doors that opened were disappointing, of course. It was a day of extremes. For every Sen. Patty Murray, there was a Sen. Mike Lee, who expressed a sick interest in the gory details of the 9/11 recovery efforts, taking no energy to pretend he cared about our health. As responders described the horrors of the recovery efforts, the equipment they'd lacked, the illnesses they'd contracted as a result, he got increasingly excited. He interrupted to ask questions like, "So you could you smell burning flesh?

What did it smell like?" with an almost gleeful twinkle in his eye, like a mischievous small child being allowed to watch a violent movie for the first time.

The speakers were taken aback by his tone. They stammered in answering, trying to stay on target. "It smelled worse than anything you can imagine." "It was like a horror movie."

Everybody who was in that meeting with Senator Lee remembers it as a watershed moment. There have been lots of times that people were dishonest with us on the Hill but very few moments where anybody was as openly delighted by the experience of watching a lineup of sick heroes rehash the details of sifting through human remains and other horror-movie-esque imagery. It made an impact. (Mike Lee, of course, was one of the only two senators to vote against the second Zadroga extension in 2019. Surprise, surprise.) Later, Rep. Steve Scalise, the GOP's Majority Whip in the House, invited us into his office and proudly showed off his collection of important documents from the Founding Fathers. He took a small private meeting with Stewart and Feal and left the rest of us to sit awkwardly in his waiting room, never to be heard from.

Despite those disappointments, other doors opened that were pretty great. At one point we were led into a conference room to wait for some mysterious guests to arrive only to watch half of the Democratic senators parade through. I took a picture with my favorite politician of the moment, Sen. Elizabeth Warren (D-MA). Sen. Cory Booker (D-NJ) snubbed me in his fist-pounding rounds, probably mistaking me for a staffer, and I've held that against him ever since. Senator Schumer made the rounds as well, gladhanding his way across the room (he, unlike Senator Booker, did not ignore my outstretched hand). Senator after senator came through to thank us for our work. Then, if that wasn't exciting enough, at the very end of the day we were ushered over to the Capitol, where we were led into a large and very ornate conference room to wait for then House Minority Leader Nancy Pelosi (D-CA) herself.

We've all seen Leader Pelosi on television or in the newspaper, some-times not in a flattering light, other times staring down groups of towering Trumpian men in a blaze of glory. Democrats and Republicans alike love to hate her. Sometimes I do too.

It's different to be in a room with her. Much as with Hillary Clinton, another female powerhouse, there is something very special about sitting next to Nancy Pelosi. I have never met anybody who radiates the kind of raw power she does, and certainly not anybody my size and similarly burdened with the many complications that come with being female in an environment defined by male power. She may be small in stature, but she has the power to alter the very atmosphere of a room just by walking into it.

Pelosi led a discussion of the Democratic strategy for the renewal bill, assuring us that it would pass and that the discussions around it and GOP demands were more theater and formality than legitimate roadblocks. For me, it was fascinating to watch. It was one of the first times in my years of work on the issue that I had ever found myself sitting in the main meeting—the one where politicians talk openly and honestly about what's going on with the people responsible for executing the public strategy. It was also a master class in how to command a room full of men. Celebrity men, big, macho, heroic responder men. It was riveting. In my regular, non-advocate life, I had been working in environments where I was talked over, ignored, or sidelined regularly. At that very moment my main profes-sional responsibilities literally involved making luxury travel arrangements and organizing meal deliveries for a male boss four years younger than me. In my prior job—the "job" job—I had been overlooked for a major promotion for being too "immature" after (or, let's be honest, because) I'd made complaints about gendered treatment at work. While I was job hunting on the heels of that experience, people consistently recommended I take entry-level positions, feigning shock at learning that I had ten years of experience under my belt because I looked so "young." (Women are never the right age in the workplace. We're always too young or too old for the job.) I was going through every day consumed by a low-grade feminist rage. That meeting with Nancy Pelosi gave me something I needed to continue slogging through the never-ending parade of casual disregard that eats away at women in so many professional environments and so much of life. It's a rare thing to experience in the flesh, but Nancy Pelosi is a behemoth. She did not invite that kind of dynamic, so nobody had the guts to create it. Even John Feal, whose success was largely related to his brash, macho messaging and leadership, was unusually quiet.

At the end of the meeting I asked Rep. Nadler to introduce me to Leader Pelosi, and his staff dutifully documented the exchange for posterity. It was glorious—the perfect ending to the most exciting twenty-four hours of my life. When I had approached the Capitol that morning, I was giddy with excitement because there was an outside chance that I'd get a picture with Jon Stewart. That was as big as I could dream. I didn't know Nancy Pelosi was even in the offing.

IN EARLY DECEMBER I returned to New York for yet another STAC meeting—a surprising two in one year! I basked in my usual nameplate glory while listening to some of those dreaded PowerPoint presentations, but the timing was ideal, because two days later I boarded another train for DC. Another lobbying adventure was planned, and HHC once again bought me and a few other survivor advocates train tickets. This time the trip was to attend a press conference at the Capitol urging members of Congress to schedule a vote on the Zadroga renewal legislation. The vote seemed imminently likely. Jon Stewart was back and gave a speech. Carole King was invited to speak about her family connections to the FDNY and broke into the national anthem but forgot the words, forcing us all into a very awkward situation since our straight, solemn faces were needed to project the seriousness of the situation, and yet it was nearly impossible not to laugh. (Jon Stewart did not. I may have giggled.) At the very end, a survivor from Battery Park City gave brief remarks.

It took me a while to read the winds, but this day felt different from September. Chillier. Responder advocates and our supposed political allies seemed to have agreed upon a strategy shift without us. As I watched most of the New York delegation members speak, I noticed that a majority didn't mention the survivor community anywhere in their remarks. Of the five or six politicians who spoke, only Rep. Nadler said anything about the people of Lower Manhattan. As we stood around in the background of the presser crowd, hidden behind very official-looking men in uniforms, a feeling of discomfort began to creep over me. I noticed looks of concern slowly sneaking onto the faces of other survivor advocates as well. Nobody seemed happy to see us; nobody on the political side was making eye contact. When the press conference was over and we tried to head inside with the responder lobbying teams, we asked staffers where we should report. They were evasive. Finally, Kimberly Flynn of 9/11 Environmental Action spoke to one of the event's coordinators. The rest of us stood around awkwardly, waiting to hear whether we'd taken a three-hour train trip that morning for nothing. His answer, relayed via Kimberly, was that we weren't invited to lobby. We were, in fact, not to visit any offices. We were told it would be detrimental to the cause.

I didn't respect that reasoning. Being allowed to advocate for yourself in the halls of Congress isn't an invite-only thing. We hadn't agreed to disappear. We hadn't been consulted on a strategy shift. We, too, were stakeholders. It was a moment that summed up perfectly all my old lines about why I've never gone to work in politics. As much as I enjoy the empowering feeling of advocating for myself, I never want to be the person who tells a group of traumatized people that telling their story is less important than protecting somebody else's, in this case the responders', image. I don't know what had changed from that September, what made survivors suddenly dangerous to the success of the bill. What conversations I wasn't privy to after I left Nancy Pelosi's office that day. It was clear, however, that the agreed-upon strategy no longer involved us.

At the most basic level, what I most took issue with was the assertion that we were detrimental to our own cause. I knew that I was an effective communicator. I had seen how impactful I could be in a lobbying meeting. I understood the political realities of the situation, that on the Hill this was about money, not strictly about helping people, but I didn't think that was a good enough excuse to tell me that my community's needs weren't important enough to speak about. Though it had been strongly implied at times in the past, that day was the first time I was directly told to sit back and ride responder coattails and not complain. I did not like it, especially after the high of that day in September. Survivors were, as always, the group most likely to see cuts in the legislation aimed at them. That was specifically because our story wasn't well understood on the Hill or by the public. That's what happens when it's implicitly understood that for every four respond-ers who get to speak to a room full of staffers, only one nonresponder survivor will be invited (if that many), when the total affected population has an estimated three to four times more survivors than responders.[221] It's what happens when all medical research is done exclusively on a subset of the disaster population that is almost 90 percent male,[222] leaving women without the stats to show how their health has been impacted nor coverage for those conditions. It's what happens when your own representatives take care not to mention your existence in their remarks to the press.

Whether or not the bill's sponsors promised that these cuts wouldn't happen was irrelevant because if we weren't in the room, we weren't going to know what kinds of compromises were on the table. We were being asked to trust a process we had no reason to trust, yet the staffers and strategists kicking us out of the room were also people we needed to cooperate with so that they'd feel enough goodwill toward us to deliver on their promise of protecting our funding. We were in a tough spot, and we'd essentially come to DC for nothing, and yet I was still high off the glory of that day in September so, in my youthful optimism, I proposed we go rogue.

I've never seen that very tenacious group of community advocates—people who have again and again gone to the mat defending me or protecting other community members from arbitrary and confusing policy defeats, people who made their bones chasing the EPA out of various downtown events—so crushed. Only one of the five or so we'd traveled with took me up on my offer to lead them on a rogue congressional adventure. I promised we wouldn't do anything that would compromise the bill, but I reminded them that I had come from California, where the reps were not hearing about this issue every day, and told them that if we wanted to protect our place in the bill we could at least lobby other supportive Democrats who might not be aware of the intricacies of the issue. We could let them know to keep an eye out for us. We started with California senator Barbara Boxer's office and made our way to as many states as we could that had StuyHealth members living in them.

We didn't ruin anything. The bill did wind up passing as part of an omnibus bill, renewing funding for the WTC Health Program for seventy-five years, making that program effectively permanent. It only extended the VCF for another five years, however—that ended up being the compromise cut.[223] The legislation passed in the House by 316–113 and was approved in the Senate, despite 33 opposition votes.[224] The president signed it into law by that Friday, December 18, 2015.[225]

That press conference at which we were pushed aside was depicted in every news story about the passage, a now famous shot of Jon Stewart, flanked by Sen. Kirsten Gillibrand and Rep. Carolyn Maloney. I'm just off to the left, as I am in so many of the iconic shots in this struggle: perpetually too short, not famous enough, and always with a dash of "mistaken for a staffer."

I understand why survivors and community members got sidelined sometimes. I know we complicate the issue because then it's no longer about heroes and wartime patriotism, it's about caring for regular people and government lies. Still, being in the shot matters because being in the memory matters. In the years since 2010 and 2015 I've spent a lot of time asserting to other advocates, all of whom are much older than me, much bigger than me, and who think of themselves as much more experienced than me, that I was there, wherever "there" is. It's important I continually reassert myself because when people conveniently forget that I was in the room for the iconic moments of this struggle, they sometimes try to tell me a different story about what happened in that room. If you ask anybody today, survivors were never told we couldn't lobby at any point in the Zadroga funding process. Responders will sometimes even suggest to me that we just don't seem to care as much. That we're not as serious as they are about the issue. That we must not be very sick. (That's code for we must not be very deserving.) At the time the numbers supported that because, of the seventy-one thousand people getting care at the WTC Health Program, only about eight thousand were survivors.[226] What nobody ever mentioned was that responders automatically get monitoring and program membership, even if they aren't sick. Survivors have to be sick with something from a very specific list of conditions to even sign up. Unsurprisingly, women's and developmental health conditions are not well represented on that list, meaning women and children are less likely to qualify for monitoring in the first place.

Sometimes I have to even remind myself that I *was* there, that my eyes saw what they saw even if nobody noticed them watching. Bearing witness is a part of my job as an advocate too.

CHAPTER 11

COMING FORWARD

The outreach work continued, but as the end of 2017 rolled around, my career was once again in flux and my advocacy work had to take a back seat. The TV show I'd been working on got canceled, and my boss started a production company. I was kept on and given a raise and a new title, but it quickly became clear that the whole exercise was an elaborate bid to keep me from quitting my assistant role during a time of great transition. I'd been hoping and prepping for a creative role, and I tried to be proactive about promoting my creative skills, but nothing seemed to stick. I gave notes on things nobody wanted notes on, I did rewrites on things I was never going to be credited for, and I worked hard to get face time with people and set up an office on the Fox Lot, hoping to retain the flexibility but not the isolation of working from home. In the middle of all that change, I got a call from a reporter looking for a survivor to speak about their experience with a 9/11-linked cancer. Cancer and 9/11: an evergreen story in the New York press. Must have been a slow news week. I gave them a name.

A good friend of mine from high school, Michele, had suffered from a series of bizarre health issues in her twenties, among them thyroid cancer. She believed her issues were related to 9/11 but had been hesitant about speaking out and opening herself up to the media's morbid fascination with serious illness. In late 2017, however, I suspected she might be interested because she was about to publish a book about the ways in which gender and illness intersect.[227] When I called her about the opportunity, I suggested that she might be able to use the press around her 9/11 health concerns to publicize the book. Opportunistic? Maybe, but good for both her and the survivor community. She hesitantly agreed, and I forwarded her information to the reporter. In mid-November she found her face plastered across the *New York Post* with the salacious headline "Cancer Cluster at Top NYC School near Ground Zero, Grad Says."[228] Other press picked up the story, and suddenly there were stories running in local, national, and international media. Advocates and reporters alike began asking if I could get more young victims to come forward, and into the middle of this, the United Federation of Teachers (UFT) arrived.

The UFT was an interesting case. They are New York's chapter of the American Federation of Teachers and represent most of the city's public school teachers, as well as other school staff positions. On and after 9/11, all of Stuyvesant's teachers belonged to the UFT, but for years they'd been absent from the 9/11 survivor discussion. When their chief of staff, a cancer survivor, learned about the Victim Compensation Fund for the first time, and found out that she qualified for a payout and that many of their members would as well, she singlehandedly changed their tune and insisted they pour a bunch of resources into getting the word out.[229] Suddenly they were everywhere, looking to make up for lost time. In late 2017 they floated the idea of putting on an informational forum at Stuyvesant High School, and StuyHealth was invited to cosponsor. We accepted, along with 9/11 Environmental Action and a VCF law firm that had been doing informational outreach as well, Barasch McGarry Salzman & Penson.

The new influx of resources was exciting, but there were some familiar obstacles as well. The UFT had the will and a sophisticated press operation, Barasch had the money, but nobody seemed to have any real sense of what they were up against when it came to finding survivor speakers to tell their stories. For the most part, they'd seen survivors appear in the papers in the past and assumed it would be easy to get others to step forward. Unfortunately, it's always been incredibly hard.

As we dove into the planning for our event, I began to ask about speakers. Everybody at the UFT assured me that they had the speakers covered. Then, as the date grew closer, they started asking me to see if any students I knew could speak about being a patient at the WTC Health Program or a VCF claimant. Alongside their speakers, of course. Just to give another perspective. When we finally showed up at the press conference before the event, StuyHealth members were the only patients there. One of the unchanging challenges of advocating for the survivor community has always been that survivors, by and large, do not like to speak to press.

Coming forward with an illness is a fraught process. I know because I've done it, not with cancer but with a list of frustratingly unsexy diseases like GERD, asthma, and PTSD. Identifying yourself as somebody in frail health, somebody worthy of sympathy, isn't enjoyable, and after an event like 9/11, the feeling that in coming forward you're claiming some sort of special victimhood makes the decision to do it even harder. Many of us in the survivor world never got validation in the first place that in showing up at school, at home, or at work we were doing something courageous, or at least dangerous and worthy of public interest. We had to actively work to forget how much courage it took just to move on with our lives after 9/11 and not stew in anger and fear. Asking us to own this feeling, to come forward and claim it, is a big ask.

Alongside that concern is the fact that everybody in the 9/11 community worries about accidentally diminishing people's sense of loss from that day itself, especially those who lost family members, colleagues, and friends. That concern is not paranoia. I've spoken to many responders who feel awkward seeking help because they survived after losing colleagues and friends in the initial collapse. Even my own friends feel it, sometimes at the hands of family members who weren't there or other contacts who aren't familiar with their story. In 2019 a friend in California, the spouse of a Stuyvesant classmate of mine, told me that, for years, she'd been thinking my work on 9/11 health issues was wildly insensitive. "I lost an uncle that day," she told me. "You didn't lose anybody." Her husband, my former classmate, had been quietly worrying about his health anyway, finding that concern difficult to vocalize. As soon as she understood, he raised concerns about his own health, asking if exposure to the air at Ground Zero might explain why his whole body is so reactive, why he has weird allergy symptoms and unexplained rashes and stomachaches. I'd like to say my friend's change of heart was instigated by exciting news about my work or my appearances in Congress and on the news, but it was unfortunately the death of another Stuy alum from a 9/11-linked cancer that opened the door for her. After that, she could see that we had both lost people. It's easy to see the victims as a limited, singular group confined to the day itself, harder to understand the attacks as a continuum that did kill people in 2001 and will continue to do so. In my experience, people from outside of New York seem to especially struggle with this knowledge.

There are other challenges for survivors in coming forward as well, like worries about what legal standard a health claim needs to meet to go to press. People coming forward for the first time often aren't very familiar with the research findings that back up their experiences, so they sometimes feel they are overdramatizing the connection between their illness and the WTC cleanup or misleading the public by making that connection. It's a fair concern—they are, after all, being asked to claim something inherently unprovable. There is no way to make a specific connection between 9/11 and an illness diagnosed years later, plus nobody can ever say definitively, in any situation, that the cause of a cancer is one particular event or exposure. It's always more complicated than that. The Zadroga Act's presumption is not that the WTC cleanup was the sole definitive cause of anybody's illness but that having WTC exposure increased a person's risk of getting sick.[230] That distinction, between presumption and proof, is not always well understood.

Our health care system doesn't make any of this easier. Survivors and responders face an inherent risk in going public with a preexisting condition thanks to our confusing patchwork of health insurance laws. Though coverage for people with prior health issues is protected by federal policy for the moment, Americans are in constant danger of losing these protections.[231] For many survivors, especially those of us who don't get benefits through a job and purchase insurance in the individual marketplace, this is a real concern. As I've mentioned, after the early publicity around my 9/11-related health concerns, none of which are life-threatening but all of which are chronic, I couldn't buy health insurance in California. It was part of why I took my "job" job—I had to desperately search around for a stable insurance option in the form of a career move. Millions of people are in the same boat, some with no job to rescue them. An estimated 54 million Americans have a preexisting condition that would have been "declinable" in the pre-ACA insurance market, and more than twice that number have conditions that would have triggered additional costs or specific coverage denials before the law changed.[232] And even in 2019, before the COVID crisis caused millions of people to lose their employer-sponsored insurance,[233] almost 50 Americans were either independently insured or uninsured, meaning they didn't have the protections of employer or federal health plans, which will often cover people regardless of their health history.[234] A slew of very boring, very technical, seemingly ephemeral insurance regulations can become life-or-death matters to survivors and others with preexisting conditions. For people who remember the pre-2014 insurance market, it's easy to see a risk in speaking up.

Finally, and perhaps most importantly, anybody who comes forward, responder or survivor, comes up against the larger American distrust of people who admit to needing public services. After many decades of politicians stigmatizing welfare recipients and others receiving public funding, beginning long before 1976, when Ronald Reagan introduced the concept of the "welfare queen" into modern parlance,[235] it's no surprise (though it remains disappointing) that many people are suspicious of any kind of community in need.[236] The list of qualities that make somebody worthy of help in the eyes of many Americans isn't straightforward, but though responders and survivors both get pushback rooted in this issue, there is an interesting distinction in how. Nobody wants to go on the record opposing care for 9/11 responders. Behind closed doors, when responders asked for funding, though politicians griped about it and dragged their feet in a completely unacceptable way, public and political opposition was generally expressed by deflecting to a conversation about money and cost. Questioning whether responders inherently deserved the help was rightfully unacceptable. When the downtown community asked for assistance, opponents articulated their concerns differently. They didn't just talk about cost; they questioned what we did to deserve the money in the first place. The way distinctions between survivors and responders were made and so readily accepted by the public is related to how our government and our media discuss need and deservingness more broadly. The language used to discuss survivors often felt like it was designed to make us look greedy instead of worthy. That's because it was.

Like my friend's wife who lost an uncle on 9/11, the opponents of funding survivor care quietly doubted we had done anything dangerous enough to be worthy of the help. Instead we were treated to stories of fraudsters like Tania Head, an early survivor advocate whose story of surviving the attacks from the 78th floor of the World Trade Center turned out to be fraudulent,[237] meant to stir up memories of the many (imaginary) welfare queens before her.

ALONG WITH THE UFT event planned for the following February, late 2017 brought other complicating dynamics as well, chief among them a sudden influx of law firm money. A cadre of personal injury firms that specialized in workers' comp claims for the city's fire and police unions had built a good business in representing people on their VCF claims. It is a volume business—attorney fees are capped at 10 percent in the Zadroga legislation,[238] which is far less than the 30 to 40 percent contingent fees that personal injury attorneys generally work with,[239] so VCF firms are constantly doing outreach to potential new clients. Most of the firms had been working on this issue for years, but without the distraction of the health program needing renewal, they suddenly had an opportunity to run with the VCF expiration messaging. They wanted to get the VCF renewed, but they also wanted to get as much business as possible before the five years of funding were up in 2020. That meant finding new customers, and for some firms, that meant turning to the survivor community for the first time.

Beginning in late November 2017, a handful of firms began setting up informal calls or meetings about how we might work together and how their resources might be useful in helping us, the survivor advocates, do our work. After years of focusing primarily on the responder community, they began turning up more visibly at events geared toward survivors, setting up tables at town halls and recruiting advocates from the nonprofit side to run outreach offices for them. They were frustrated by the careful approach the groups working under NIOSH's federal outreach contracts, groups like mine, were using to get the word out. As federal contractors, we had to be incredibly careful not to spread disinformation, even if by accident. We had specific language we could use to describe the health program (care was "no cost," not "free," because for survivors the program would cover only the costs insurance didn't pick up, not the entire bill for services) and specific ways we organized events, which always included as many "official" representatives of the programs as possible. Even when those official people gave boring presentations or were combative with the audience, we had to suffer through to keep our funding.

The personal injury world is, in a word, different. It's the Wild West. Their advertising budget was largely spent on alarming mailers and a familiar kind of commercial—complete with a stern voice announcing that if you or a loved one went through such-and-such event and got cancer you may be entitled to money, stark graphics, the serious faces of a roomful of people in expensive suits ready to "fight for you," and an air of parody. By late 2018, people in Lower Manhattan were being blanketed with mail, television ads, and radio commercials advertising free money, all consistently repeating the refrain that they could get cancer from 9/11. The panic it was driving in the community certainly made people more receptive to our less splashy work on the federal contractor side, but it also meant that anybody trying to advertise a Zadroga program, whether or not it enriched them financially, was tarnished by the somewhat seedy reputation of the personal injury world. No matter who we were, we were being perceived as potentially crooked by a growing percentage of our audience.

The private money also meant that there was a lot of incomplete and incorrect information flowing around, and this suddenly became our problem too. Just as we had wrongly considered the VCF a secondary program for years—something we only recommended to people who were gravely ill—the VCF attorneys were fairly disinterested in the WTC Health Program beyond its role in certifying conditions for the VCF. That meant that they were driving a lot of people to that program, sometimes overwhelming the health program's intake process, but weren't letting their clients know much about the treatment services it offered.

Most of these VCF firms, financial incentives aside, were well intentioned. A lot of them, in fact, were located in Lower Manhattan and staffed by survivors themselves. Many had come to work just after 9/11 and cleaned up their offices in dangerous conditions. Many had gotten sick as a result, so they intrinsically understood the fear the community was feeling.

What the lawyers didn't always understand, however, having worked primarily with responders up until that point, was how survivors are treated differently by the health program. How they can't sign up to be monitored without already being sick. Why this makes our outreach work complicated and slow and sometimes ineffective. They would get impatient with us as we insisted on clarity in their advertising, hoping to avoid sending survivors to their one free screening appointment without all the facts, and at other times they simply gave survivors incorrect information about who qualified for care. They had a louder voice than us because of the money and no federal overlords, so they could do as they pleased.

I HAD ALREADY BEEN approaching one of my periodic phases of 9/11 burnout when the conversation about how the survivor community would interact with these lawyers came up ahead of the UFT's event. Listening to people's traumatic stories is draining. Holding their hands through paperwork dramas is exhausting. I'd also, perhaps as a part of my post-2015 anxiety, been feeling diminished—deferring to other people and approaching other advocates and organizers as if I was just lucky to be invited along. I entered 2018 hesitant to raise issues, quick to apologize if I got rebuffed. I allowed myself to be left out of the loop at critical moments. My uncertainty had consequences, as other people began to take credit for my press work. I allowed myself to be treated like I was inexperienced, and I allowed organizations and new partners to explain things to me that were related to my own areas of expertise. I allowed the UFT and Barasch McGarry and all of our other event partners in that February event to approach the planning as if nobody had ever thought or tried to do outreach to schools when I had a decade of experience doing it. I started to feel smaller and smaller, working harder and harder for less and less benefit. It was an experience that paralleled the moment I was having in my career in Hollywood, where I was also doing more and more for less and less credit. I was running out of energy to combat it all.

I only noticed I was shrinking because 9/11 Environmental Action's director, Kimberly Flynn, began to see it. She acted as my Sherpa and cheerleader, as she often has in these moments. She called me a few days before the UFT event and, in her characteristically wordy way (calls with her are famous for never ending, for morphing into a full rundown of everything on her mind), told me to make more demands. To get my logo onto the poster. Get my name into the press. "Are they giving you a speaking spot? They're talking about students but they don't know any of them. They don't have an event without you." She repeatedly reminded me that I was a "get." That I was not just lucky to be contacted by people with the resources to do outreach but was an effective advocate with a track record of convincing other students to actually speak out. Sometimes I wonder why I still need somebody to remind me of my value at times it should be obvious, but then I remember that this feeling is by design. It serves people in power, whatever level of power that is, for those of us doing the boring, unglamorous work to feel like we can't ask for credit when that credit is due. It's something that every young advocate has to learn to ignore at some point, but it's not easy.

Getting the full benefits of participation took more than cheerleading, of course. On the way to the event, Kimberly also had the unenviable task of letting me know that I couldn't use StuyHealth's name in the press outreach around the event. The feds had decided that the presence of a VCF lawyer made it inadvisable for their contractors to attend. Three of my Stuyvesant classmates and I spoke at the press conference before the forum, along with Kimberly Flynn, the head of the UFT, and Michael Barasch from the law firm Barasch McGarry. Though I'd been assuming the other organizations were bringing speakers because that's what I'd been told, Kimberly had suspected otherwise, and she was right. All of the patient stories had come through my work. I'd recruited the classmates individually, messaging every person who'd ever contacted me with questions about the WTC Health Program or VCF, either via Facebook or via email, asking if they'd be willing to speak to the public about their experience. A young cancer survivor said she'd be happy to. Two asthmatic classmates of mine agreed to talk about their experience with the program. In between the press conference and the event, the four of us sat down to lunch at one of the few still-operating diners near the school. We'd all spent a lot of time there as teenagers, munching on french fries with our different crowds of friends. I revisited a classic, if not eccentric, order of mine: chicken soup and a side of fries. They were salty and delicious. The weather was frigid so I ordered a hot chocolate too and we chuckled about how some of us never grow up. After a morning of 9/11 talk, it only took an hour or two to return to a scene of happier high school memories.

GIVEN THE HAPHAZARD NATURE of the planning process, I wasn't surprised when the event itself turned out to be sparsely attended. The UFT had promised people would just "show up," but survivors never do that. Survivors often don't realize they count as an affected population in the first place.

With the focus squarely on the VCF, the tone of the event was a little different from what I was used to. At forums involving only the WTC Health Program, the information is usually about procedure and care, not about how to overcome your guilt about using the program. People have to be sick to be in the survivor program, and anybody who isn't is generally only asking about procedure because they worry they'll become sick.

The tone is, as it turns out, very different when the service being featured is not care for a diagnosed health issue but a pile of money. The other speakers kept repeating a refrain about how, if people felt too guilty about getting money from the Victim Compensation Fund, they should file a claim anyway and donate the money to charity. It's a popular talking point with responder audiences, and the exhortation was primarily coming from people with little experience speaking to the survivor community. For those of us used to working on the community side, it rubbed us the wrong way.

In the survivor community we often focus on procedure with the implication that everybody should already know we deserve the care. We don't ever echo media messages that make it seem like we didn't do something in the aftermath of the attacks to make us worthy of services—we hear that enough. Suggesting that people should donate their compensation money to charity undercuts the message that we fight for—that we exist, that we are worthy—by suggesting that we might, or should, feel "guilty" about getting a payout, as if it's money that we don't actually deserve. This guilt messaging was a new obstacle, one we hadn't thought to worry about but vowed to learn from since it was looking like the VCF, either its upcoming expiration or renewal, were going to become a major focus of our work for the next year.

For my part, as they handed the microphone to me, I found that I was so distracted by the new talk of dollars and guilt that my usual talking points didn't feel like they would suffice. Instead I dug deep and found the long-buried side of me that's a little bit of a ham. I smiled. I made jokes. The pictures from the event are notable because my posture is all sass. My face looks mid–punch line in every photo, like I'm just about to laugh at my own joke somewhere in a monologue about young adults and illness. At the same time, I reiterated: "We were all here. We all breathed in the air. We all have access to the health program and VCF. These programs are for us too." The room seemed more agitated than anything else.

Later, my expression contorted into one of teary-eyed avoidance, sparked by a moment of kismet in the auditorium. On the far side of the theater, an usher handed out a mic during the Q&A and I saw Anetta Luczak, the teacher who had evacuated with me on 9/11, get up to ask a question. Her question wasn't about the program; it was about whether I remembered that we had evacuated together. I immediately felt my eyes well up and focused on my thumbs to keep from bursting into tears. This was the first time we'd seen each other since my graduation back in 2002. She looked the same. I felt the same. As soon as we were done, I ran over to give her a hug and suddenly the UFT newsletter's photographer was all over us. By that point I had stopped being self-conscious about the tears. I was just so happy to see her.

EMBARRASSINGLY ENOUGH, THAT FEBRUARY event was
where I learned that I, too, qualified for the VCF. Clearly part of my
bewilderment at the change in outreach tone was because I, like much of
the survivor community, had never quite overcome the assumption that it
was for responders only. I knew it intellectually, but it didn't *feel* like it was
for me. Then, after the influx of lawyer advertising, I promptly plunged my
head in the sand and left it there.

My longtime confusion was largely related to the fund's history. The
original VCF was established just after 9/11 to provide compensation to
people injured in the attacks and to the families of the victims who died
on the day, and something of that reputation had stuck with me. That
fund closed in 2004, having distributed over $7 billion to the families of
the more than 2,880 people who died on 9/11 and the more than 2,500
injured on the day.[240] When Congress reopened the fund in 2011, the focus
was different. Now a part of the Zadroga Act, the VCF was authorized to
provide benefits to sick and injured responders and survivors as well.[241]
Still, since political opponents had raised (largely insincere) concerns about
fraud,[242] there were lots of rules, and the special master at the time didn't
make them any clearer.

Everybody else on the advocacy side seemed similarly unsure about
where the survivor community fit into the regulations, and the Justice
Department,[243] which manages the program, had spent years giving survivors the impression that we were discouraged from applying. It had worked.
Those few classmates with serious illnesses had gotten payouts; survivors in
general, especially those with less critical conditions, felt it wasn't their place
to apply because *what if the fund ran out of money before every responder
could access it and it became* our fault *that some poor responder family was
going without? And how should survivor claimants prove that they qualify?*
Nobody seemed to be sure.

In 2016, a new special master, Rupa Bhattacharyya, was appointed. She
quickly made changes to the claim-filing process, allowing the VCF to rely

on certifications from the WTC Health Program to determine eligibility instead of a mess of private medical documents. Staff was sent to outreach events to explain program policy and encourage survivors to apply, even those with chronic but common illnesses.[244] By 2018 I knew about these changes but hadn't quite grasped that anybody with any diagnosed physical health condition from the WTC Health Program, even something like asthma, could qualify for compensation. I wasn't clear on the distinction between payouts meant to help people recoup financial losses related to their illness and "pain and suffering" payouts, which anybody who was sick could qualify for. Once I understood, it made sense—spending your twenties with a chronic health issue has many costs that you can't show receipts for.

Over dinner following the outreach event, one of the VCF attorneys from Barasch's firm set me straight, and my mind was blown. It turned out that almost every patient at the WTC Health Program (with the sole exclusion of people who are only seeking mental health care) could apply and get, at the minimum, something in the range of $20,000.[245] Even I could apply with my asthma and GERD diagnoses.[246] They offered to represent me pro bono, but warned me that the process takes years.

As of mid-2019, the VCF had awarded over $5.174 billion in compensation to nearly 22,500 claimants, but there were many more people out there still waiting for their compensation and, as we learned from that 2018 event, many more who qualified and didn't know it.[247] At the same time we were learning that the fund was running out of money—it had only been appropriated $7.375 billion between the 2011 and 2015 bills and was set to overrun that amount long before the December 18, 2020, renewal deadline, assuming, of course, that there was even a renewal.[248] By late 2018 the special master was suggesting they might have to cut award amounts (and she did a few months later in February 2019).[249] There was a new time sensitivity to applying.

BRASH LAW-FIRM TACTICS ASIDE, understanding that survivors qualified for compensation but faced a deadline was key to turning the VCF into a huge boon for our outreach work. Some people are attracted to messaging about no-cost health care, but many more are drawn to free money. Especially when they are running out of time to get it.

Though I knew that VCF deadlines were fast-approaching and outreach operations were kicking into high gear, I was surprised by what happened next. In November 2018, Barasch McGarry, the firm putting the most resources into doing survivor-focused outreach, offered me a job. In some ways, their timing was impeccable. I'd just quit my day job, the TV experience that never quite panned out, and was looking for my next move.

Still, I sensed I was facing a watershed moment in my political life, one I'd built my entire career around avoiding. I was being asked, pretty directly, to cash in the credibility I had developing with the community over the years to sell a specific VCF firm's services to potential VCF claimants. Essentially, to sell out.

It wasn't exactly on the level of going to work for Big Oil—these firms provided a useful service. And that's also not to say that the firm didn't make an appealing pitch, reminding me that advocacy doesn't pay the bills but that they could make a lot of the advocacy work I wanted to do possible. We shared a goal of getting VCF legislation renewed the following year, and my costs in participating in that work would be covered instead of being a major financial strain on me personally as they had been in the past. I'd have resources to throw into new outreach efforts as well and would be free to advertise the WTC Health Program alongside the VCF. I'd even have access to media. Taken that way, it sounded like a great deal.

I had always wondered how these moments happen, why people go for the sell-out option. I get it now. I was broke, unemployed, and scared. It was an offer that was flexible and generous, being made by somebody I knew to be a survivor himself and a dedicated advocate on the issue.

There was something that bugged me about it, though. It was the way the offer implied that the WTC Health Program outreach, which I'd been doing for next to nothing for years, was a side hustle I was running. Almost like they considered my relationship with that program to be a financial arrangement similar to what they had going with the VCF, as if I somehow personally benefited from getting customers in the door. I felt like they couldn't understand a world in which I just did the work because it was right to. Despite all their talk about how they do good work, which, to be clear, they were and are doing, they were suspicious of the idea that sometimes people do the right thing because they should—not for meaningful personal gain. They framed everything in a very transactional way, brushing off slightly unethical suggestions as if they were a cost of doing business, frustrated that I wanted to stay on good terms with my most tireless cheerleader, Kimberly, and the others I'd been working with for more than a decade.

I've made bad choices at points in the advocacy process. I've failed my classmates and the Lower Manhattan community at times. Those failures have always been honest mistakes, though. I've never failed them because I owed somebody else a different outcome. The concerns that kept me from working in politics came flying back to me, hard. Being financially beholden to someone matters, even when you're ostensibly doing the right thing.

I told them I'd think about the offer, but though their resources were appealing and the offer generous, the idea of abandoning my independence as an advocate so soon before a major lobbying effort, even if I could still participate, didn't sit well. I held them off but didn't close the door entirely, knowing a moment might come where I had no financial choice.

As conflicted as I felt about turning the law firm down, Barasch McGarry's offer did do me a huge favor, one that I'll be forever grateful for given how much it changed my trajectory the following year. With a potential job in my back pocket, I had the flexibility to settle back into a routine instead of passing all my time listlessly trolling the internet for work. When you quit your job, even if you've saved for it and planned for it, people can't help but project their own circumstances onto you. A lot of my anxiety around quitting had been related to how people reacted to the news. They rushed to send me job postings for things I was overqualified for, assuming I was willing to take anything. They stared at me with sad, worried eyes, as if my insistence that I had savings was a delusion they didn't have the heart to refute. They'd direct me to job boards that had nothing to do with my areas of expertise. Whatever I said, they simply would not believe that I had prepared for the moment.

The truth was that I had prepared. My last job had been going badly for months, and I'd taken careful steps to set myself up for an eventual departure, knowing I might not have the chance to jump to another job immediately. I was unsure of when my departure would happen but positive it was approaching. When the end finally came it was because my boss broke a major promise that left me without any viable advancement opportunities. I wasn't fired; I quit. It was painful, but I remained confident in the decision . . . right up until I told somebody about it. I'm not a risk-taker by nature. I don't enjoy roller coasters. I carefully save from each paycheck. I use two checking accounts so that my rent money never gets spent on something silly by accident. When left to my own devices I usually make a safe choice. Still, as soon as somebody reacted to the news, projecting their own cavalier choices onto mine, I immediately forgot that I should trust myself. I started to panic about my "career" and "future" and whether the practical considerations I'd already made were sufficient.

Having that job in my back pocket helped me focus on other things, and there were lots of things to focus on that year. The VCF announced it was running out of money in 2019; its funding would be depleted in months, not years. It was also the year that many in the survivor community began to ask questions about the VCF for the first time and realize that we qualified for compensation. That year the VCF announced that, for the first time, new survivor claims were outpacing new responder claims by a significant margin.[250] It was also the year that the FealGood Foundation and other advocates decided we'd be renewing the VCF. Without a job, I was suddenly very available to participate.

CHAPTER 12

COMPENSATION

I ring in the New Year in Washington, DC, every year. I have for over a decade. I am not exactly a creature of habit, but I am a creature of custom, and I like to start and end the year the same way. I like to be with the same people, enjoying the same memories, celebrating long, loyal friendships born at Stuyvesant, no matter what is going on in my life. Also, I like to be on time. California gets to the New Year late—three hours of waiting, with the ball already dropped and Dick Clark's replacement long tucked into bed. It's brutal. Also brutal? Spending the night just a few blocks south of the horrible Times Square bonanza, where my parents live and where I usually pass the week following Christmas to make sure I catch my mother's late December birthday. DC is more sedate. The kind of place that you can spend an entire evening out and about and miraculously find yourself in your bed, pajamas on, teeth brushed, by 1:00 a.m. Sometimes it also confers lobbying benefits.

In January 2019, my DC New Year's tradition meant that I'd be in town for the first day of a new, very buzzy, very young Congress. I knew that 2019 would be the year we'd be pushing for the 9/11 Victim Compensation Fund's renewal, knew I might find myself down there again in a considerably less footloose and fancy-free position, so I decided to make some drop-in visits. I walked up to the House office buildings as the freshman members were gathering, just in time to see the newly elected Rep. Ayanna Pressley of Massachusetts, one of the more buzzy, progressive winners in the November elections, bound up to two other female freshmen and exclaim, "I can't believe we're actually here!" Like it was the first day of school. Like there were still reasons to feel optimistic, even though two years of Donald Trump as president had thrown half of the nation into a state of emotional and political disarray. It felt like a new start, and a much-needed one at that.

The optimism in the air was largely rooted in the fact that the Democrats had flipped over forty seats in the House and were welcoming more than one hundred new members into the caucus. These changes included the election of a new Democratic Congress member representing Staten Island, generally a stronghold of support for the 9/11 community even under Republican leadership, and some seats in upstate New York that are popular with NYC retirees and a growing number of millennials looking for affordable housing. I reached out to the transition teams of as many of the new Congress members as I could. One was a campaign my parents had been involved in, and they took my early-bird request very seriously. I was their office's first meeting, held in a barren room in the Longworth Building on the day after their boss was sworn in, only a skeleton staff even hired. I dropped in on the rest of the offices as they threw parties celebrating their new jobs with deli platters, schmoozing small-time donors, lobbyists flitting between offices like hummingbirds. Some of the parties were more popular than others. Some of the new staffers were more flustered than others. It was all good insight.

Having learned back in 2010 and 2015 that my role in the lobbying process was twofold—that I had the secret burden of lobbying both congressional staffers and our own advocates in hopes they'd retell our story in their meetings—I kept these early-bird meetings a secret. The VCF legislation hadn't been introduced yet, and my meetings were not really about the bill as much as they were a rogue attempt to inform potentially supportive offices about an aspect of the 9/11 health issue they might not hear much about going forward—the survivor community. As it was during my stealthy solo lobbying in 2015, my goal was mostly harm reduction. When offices from swing and conservative districts began looking for ways to make cuts to the cost of the legislation, I wanted an army of Congress members to tell them that survivors weren't the right place to look for those reductions.

It was all very theoretical, of course, since there was no actual legislation yet. I wasn't even sure how people outside New York City would react to this round of the Zadroga funding fight. The VCF is complicated to explain. It isn't something tangible like health care or prescription drugs; the fund is financial payouts made in exchange for something inherently impossible to appraise: a person's quality of life, or the cost of a life to a person's family.[251] Who can say what a fair value on that is?

I quietly made my rounds anyway, assuming I'd have limited opportunities to weave survivors into the story told later by the more famous advocates—the big-gun, press-generating players like John Feal and Jon Stewart. I figured I'd have few chances to answer the real question on many staffers' minds, which was, "You don't really think deserve as much as the responders, do you?"

I get asked this question a lot, worded just as harshly, often by people who have no background in the issue and no knowledge of Lower Manhattan's 9/11 experience. I used to answer it by talking in circles because that's what public perception demanded, but I now answer confidently with, "Yes, I do." Not as a means of denigrating the role of the responders, who have been our compatriots in this fight for years, but to remind people that a government-level lie about a community's safety is not less dangerous to some people than it is to others.

I wasn't interested in reliving 2015's diminishment of the survivor narrative. In 2019 I was ready to play offense, even if I was alone. Hopped up on some of the resentments and frustrations of the last renewal fight,

I spent that first week of the congressional session gearing up for battle, getting ready to elbow my way into the conversation. It was a little weird then, when, a few weeks after getting back to LA, I was invited by a member of Congress to pop up in DC. I was invited, in fact, to show up, walk over to a microphone, and speak at the press conference announcing the VCF renewal bill's introduction.

I wasn't sure who else would be there, what exactly they'd say, or what I was meant to say, but when Rep. Carolyn Maloney's office made the request I said yes. Then, naturally, I panicked.

The panic came in waves, but the first wasn't actually about the pressure to do well; it was about the cost. Not the emotional kind, the financial kind. That moral high ground I'd been standing on while I turned down the law firm job was starting to feel a little lonely.

NONPROFIT AND FEDERAL CONTRACT work is filled with land-mines. I'm frequently surprised by the activities I get in trouble for doing as a very part-time contributor to one federal outreach contract. Often these are things I would never think to check out with anybody before participating in, things that are good for outreach and important to our educational work. I had very specifically chosen not to make StuyHealth a 501(c)(3), an official nonprofit, knowing it would place limitations on our advocacy work, but in working very closely with other c3's like 9/11 Environmental Action, we'd become unofficially bound by c3 rules anyway. There was an argument that constantly reappeared about whether this meant that NIOSH, which had been paying me to work part-time under 9/11 Environmental Action's contract and covering StuyHealth's outreach costs, could place limitations on StuyHealth's or my advocacy work. They decided they could, and by 2019 I had learned the hard way what their list of banned activities included, though there were always more lurking around the bend.

Our contract with the National Institute for Occupational Safety and Health, according to their rules, precluded me from participating in political advocacy of any sort as a representative of StuyHealth. The rule was designed to avoid the appearance of a conflict of interest, since a tiny sliver of the Zadroga funding would technically enrich me personally. Their worries were not unfounded—the WTC Health Program and NIOSH (which runs the program) have always, especially during unfriendly administrations, had to worry about sudden cuts to their funding. They were, however, overzealous and put all of us on the advocacy side in an awkward bind. The only people who had the experience and reach to do the outreach work NIOSH required *were* advocates, the very people who also had the experience to do the legislative work. I remember having a phone call with Kimberly in which I said, "I only do this because I want to be an advocate for my classmates. I'll leave the NIOSH contract if that's what it takes." She replied, "I'll call them. I'll work something out." She always managed to. Before every DC event, as part of the deal Kimberly arranged, I would be warned not to identify myself as a member of StuyHealth, which was funny, because I am its founder.

In 2019, however, there was another obstacle—I was unemployed. Unfortunately, because of the NIOSH restrictions, I was not allowed to use StuyHealth funds to cover the cost of the trip to DC. Bad timing to enter a bizarre transitional period—my career obligations in that moment consisted of running a self-funded voter education website and trying to convince myself that it might lead to something productive. After turning down the law firm, and aside from taking on a few scattered freelance assignments, I hadn't found anything paid in months. Meanwhile, I was on my own for the cost of travel between LA and DC.

I was still on the relatively privileged end of this spectrum, of course. There are a lot of barriers that prevent people from engaging in serious advocacy work, from having the time to organize, to the many logistical obstacles that life places in everybody's way, to things as simple as performance anxiety, but there is also a direct financial cost tied to having an active political life. Activists working on poverty issues often bring up that communities of color, in having fewer financial resources after years of discrimination, inherently lose some ability to advocate for themselves. The wealth gap between Black and White families is startling and increasing—in 2019, Federal Reserve data showed that White families have, on average, eight times the wealth of the average Black family.[252] The fact that women make, on average, eighty-two cents on the dollar as compared to men (and the figure is far less for Black, indigenous, and Latina women)[253] has direct political consequences that compound those obstacles. Both of these chasms have widened further in the age of COVID.[254]

Advocacy work requires supplies. Advocates need computers, access to the internet, the ability to travel to meetings, the ability to print materials (like business cards, which are frequently exchanged in political meetings). Just the act of incorporating an organization so that it's capable of opening a bank account can cost hundreds of dollars.[255] Ultimately, if you want the work to grow, it helps to have relationships with potential donors, access to information about where to find grant money, and money to pay salaries. For that you need access to the informal networks that can offer these resources and informational support.

When it comes to health care advocacy, we sometimes ignore these concerns despite the issue's deep intersection with poverty and discrimination. Sometimes somebody rich steps up to fund the logistical costs of organizing, but when an issue or a community is not visible enough, not sexy enough, media and the rest of society often assume it's not worthy enough either.

When it comes to my own funding struggles, I have major advantages. I am white and middle-class; I attended prestigious schools, and I have never been in danger of losing a roof over my head, access to food, or any basic measure of security. The fact that my lack of outside funding did not prove to be intractable is, in fact, likely why it wound up being a Stuyvesant alum who could keep this fire burning for so long and not a high school student from one of the other, less famous, less opportunity-rich local public schools. I could pull together the $500, whether or not it was smart budgeting, whether or not I was unemployed, and fly myself to DC to be available to speak. It was lucky for me, sure, but the system that put me in that situation is shameful. Our perception of who deserves help is, among other things, inevitably linked to who can afford to fly across the country and ask for it inside the halls of power. I could do it, but it was a stretch. Many people can't do it at all. We've all heard the stat that 40 percent of Americans don't have the cash to cover a $400 emergency.[256] That's less than was required just to get me into the room.

In any case, though it wasn't one of my most genius financial decisions, I was able to eat the cost of going to DC, taking it out of the savings I'd careful scrapped together before leaving my job. It was a major opportunity, one I did not expect I'd get, to position the student community somewhere on the periphery of the renewal discussion and to remind the other advocates that a downtown student could make a compelling pitch for the survivor community's inclusion in these programs.

THE PRESS CONFERENCE ANNOUNCING the Never Forget the Heroes: Permanent Authorization of the September 11th Victim Compensation Fund Act (a name which would later be amended to be even longer!) was a surprisingly large event, not only because the bill's many sponsors were squeezed onto the stage but because it featured the ultimate DC power combo: a presidential candidate and a celebrity. The last presser I'd attended with that level of press interest was the one held two days after Hillary Clinton announced her candidacy for president in January 2007. The day I briefly acted as her bodyguard.

This time it was also the junior senator from New York, the VCF bill's Senate sponsor Sen. Kirsten Gillibrand, who had recently announced a presidential bid, putting her in the middle of an incredibly large field.

Flanking her on the right was Jon Stewart, rightly indignant that we had to come back again to ask for more responder money, but charming as always. He managed to squeeze a few chuckles out of a very hot, very uncomfortable press corps as he began his remarks, starting with, "Thank you very much. We only have 150 more speakers."[257]

After our 2015 day of glory I'd seen him a couple of times, always in passing, never positive he recognized me. The more time I spent around him, the more I could see that his fame was about a lot more than his being a comic or a TV host. A lot of people have hosted politically focused talk shows, been just as funny, and walked away with significantly less cachet. Jon has an intrinsic skill with something else—he's a sophisticated and talented political communicator. He made sense of the news for my entire generation in our least sophisticated but most formative years, and his clear, candid communication style is also why he's so effective as an advocate. He has a unique ability to say really pointed things about power, about Congress, about process, and about justice—things that the politicians smiling behind him know are directed at them—and make them laugh uncomfortably with him about their own hypocrisy. As celebrity advocates go, he's more than a "get." He's a rock star.

After relaxing the crowd at that February event, Jon got to the point: "We can cut through the nonsense here, everybody. This is about twelve Republicans on the Senate side."[258] Uncomfortable chuckles. "This program already exists. It's like you have a Starbucks card. We're just asking to get a little more money on it."[259]

Then, the moment that would make the news: "I'm going to say this now. Are all the cameras on me? The Trump Justice Department is doing an excellent job in administrating this program."[260] He tapped the mic dramatically to scattered applause and repeated the line. It played on every news network that night.

In the wide shots of Jon's remarks, you can see me standing politely off to the side. For me, despite that small run of local press in 2018, the

February 2019 presser was a bit of a re–coming out. It's the story of my life that a lot of the people on the Hill who saw me speak in 2006 and 2007, ran into me again in 2009 and 2010, crossed paths with me once more in 2015, read about me in the news in 2018, and caught me in the halls of Congress just a month earlier, had already forgotten me. I had learned a few things in the intervening years, however. Having the confidence of somebody in their mid-thirties, even if you're small and female and still perceived as being in your mid-twenties, is helpful. I decided 2019 was my year to end this cycle of congressional forgetfulness, and I did it by reaching back to my long-standing distaste for professional fashion. Basically, I wore jeans.

It worked like magic.

Standing in an outfit more appropriate for a Hollywood lunch than a legislative negotiation, I suddenly stood out from the Hill staffers, and though I got snubbed in the staging area by some of the bill's congressional sponsors as they glad-handed responders in their matching FealGood Foundation T-shirts, I patiently laid in wait. Soon I noticed staffers and, eventually, politicians themselves wondering who I was. They pointed me out to each other with raised brows. Others introduced themselves.

Jon's first punch line wasn't a joke. The presser was long, partly owing to the bill's many sponsors, which beyond Senator Gillibrand included Sen. Cory Gardner of Colorado, Senate Minority Leader Chuck Schumer, as well as Reps. Carolyn Maloney, Jerrold Nadler, and Peter King. My speaking slot came last, as always, more a symbolic nod to the survivor community than an opportunity to feature our story. The placement gave me time to get nervous, to calm myself down, to get nervous again, to overanalyze people's choice to bring notes or speak extemporaneously, and then to get nervous again. I had practiced my speech a few times the night before with my friend Kara, my closest childhood friend and perpetual host in DC—she's close enough to being family that she sometimes receives texts from me that I'm on the way as I sit in the airport in LA and comes home to find me sitting on her couch, eating her food, ruining her Netflix algorithm. Because I camp out at her house, she is often my coach as I nervously work my way through my preperformance rituals and her entire cupboard of snacks. The night before the presser she had given me some helpful feedback and rehearsed with me until well past midnight, when she finally mentioned it might be nice to get some sleep before work.

Kara is also a great role model for these nervous moments, but not because she acts like a best-friend character from a movie. She doesn't pepper me with inspirational sayings or tell me to take deep breaths. Sometimes she even sends me out the door with mild criticism and a nagging feeling that I should think of something better to say. Kara's power is instead that she has impossibly high standards for her friends. Since long before I met her in fourth grade, she's been aggressively confident in ways that women simply aren't supposed to be. I once pointed out that she was explaining to me how television, which is my own area of professional expertise, works. She replied, "I know a lot about a lot of things, Lila. I can't help that."

Sometimes it takes people a little while to figure out what to do with Kara's almost confrontational assuredness, but the secret is that you just have to suck it up and be confident back. Her most generous and wonderful quality is that she expects everybody to be as self-possessed as she is. She'd, in fact, prefer if everyone was. She's a loyal friend and supporter, but when I'm feeling timid or full of doubts, she doesn't calm me down by sympathizing. Instead she is totally aghast, as if she can't comprehend why I wouldn't just assume that I'm smarter and more capable than everybody else. Her pep talks come in the form of flippant comments like, "I don't know why you're worried about this. You're smarter than most people" and "These people should be taking their talking points from you, not vice versa." I leave her house hopped up on my own brilliance and ready for combat. It's the perfect preparation for the consistent scorn one faces as an advocate on the Hill.

That said, Kara's boosting can only do so much about the physical strain that comes from standing for over an hour at a press conference in a very hot room. My knees were starting to lock as I heard my name called by Senator Gillibrand, who for some reason read a bio for me that included not just my advocacy work but the very sexy facts that I suffer from asthma and GERD. Usually, unless they are introducing somebody who has been invited to speak specifically because they are a patient or got involved because of a deadly condition, people don't introduce us advocates by our health conditions at these things. Gillibrand really highlighted my illnesses, which seemed especially lame compared to the litany of cancer survivors who had spoken before me. She didn't pronounce GERD like a word, as most people do. She read the letters one by one, punctuating each letter so dramatically that people around me started to giggle.

Just walking to the podium, getting a chance to do something more than stand and stare solemnly at the cameras, was a relief, but I heard the huddle's contagious titters my whole way up there, and looking serious myself became a briefly agonizing struggle. The sheer amount of time I had spent focusing on not fainting and not getting blocked by tall people was challenge enough. I didn't need to contract a laughing fit.

Luckily, a debacle with my notes helped cure my church giggles. I had prepared some talking points, but they were on my phone, and when the phone didn't unlock, I had to abandon the idea of reading. I laid my dead phone down on the podium and started speaking extemporaneously, doing my best to hit all the points Kara and I had gone through, staring straight into a specific lens in front of me. Some of the press had cleared out by the time things got to me, and the room was starting to hum with the boredom of people who had watched too many speeches. I held my line as best I could. I mentioned that we had been put in a dangerous situation when we were not even old enough to advocate for ourselves, and for us that's not just a talking point, because that choice has made us sick.[261] I made sure they knew we were talking about serious illnesses, not just my now hilarious GERD.

"We used to hear mostly about chronic but manageable conditions that could be treated with affordable medications," I said. "We now regularly hear about students that are coming down with cancers and other serious illnesses."

"We were very young when we were exposed, so we're just starting to see our illness rates spike now, just as the VCF is about to close its doors to us. That means that classmates of mine are going to find out that they are sick years from now and they are not going to be able to access help."[262]

I soon felt the audience start to focus, and I held that focus.

"If this program is slowly drained and allowed to expire, it will be just another example of a time that we were forgotten by a government that thought it was more important that Lower Manhattan return to normal than it was to take care of the children that had experienced a major tragedy down there. This program is there to protect us. Our suffering is not going to end on a deadline. It's not going to slowly diminish by 50 to 70 percent, and so neither should this program."[263]

My speech never made it into any press. It was never my expectation that it would—after all, there were clips of Jon Stewart for the media to pull from. There were snippets of a very theatrical John Feal, still the FealGood Foundation front man and responder media darling. There were politicians to curry favor with, an opportunity for the media to give them airtime (all politicians love airtime) in exchange for access later. I measured my effectiveness as a speaker using a different metric—the speed with which Senator Schumer, the Senate Minority Leader and senator from New York, darted across the huddle to shake my hand. Like I was a bomb that needed diffusing.

SCHUMER'S RELATIONSHIP TO THE 9/11 health issue was complicated. In 2006, Kristen Lombardi, the reporter who did that first major reporting on StuyHealth, also wrote an article entitled "While Schumer Slept" in which local activists noted that he'd been notoriously absent from the 9/11 health conversation. As Lombardi wrote, "For years, he said nothing about the putrid air, or the noxious dust, or the people getting sick. It wasn't until 2006—mostly since [a mid-2006] congressional hearing—that Schumer became a consistent and visible player on the front lines of this battle."[264] My fellow survivor advocate Kimberly Flynn is quoted as saying, "When it comes to people we represent, he has been nowhere."[265] A group of Stuyvesant parents were also interviewed and decried his seemingly purposeful lack of involvement in the Stuyvesant plight, saying of his response to their attempts to get in touch with his office that "It was some form of buck passing" and "We were given the runaround continuously."[266] The piece was brutal, but despite the fact that this perception was still floating around New York, clouding his reputation, Schumer hadn't raised his head to do anything more than whip some final Senate votes during the previous Zadroga funding rounds.

I had been especially shocked by Schumer's hands-off approach to this issue when I first got involved, because his daughter was a classmate of mine at Stuyvesant. In Lombardi's piece, his staff and even his own words suggest that Schumer's hesitancy to get involved was actually *because* he was a parent at Stuyvesant on 9/11. He told Lombardi that his daughter specifically asked him not to intervene. Lombardi wrote, "When asked if he ever explained that silence to parents with growing concerns about their children's health, he replies, 'That's not the point.' He adds: 'I may not have wanted to tell them because I may have wanted to keep my daughter's situation private.'"[267] Lombardi, for her part, forever the intrepid reporter, suggested that perhaps the real reason for his silence had more to do with not wanting to contradict his wife, an official in Giuliani's city hall, who had also declared the area safe. He certainly seemed to toe the line when he walked his daughter back to school on October 9, 2001, and told reporters, "They've done all the testing,"[268] and, "I know they've made it safe."[269]

Either way, not wanting to drag a classmate into the discussion against her will, I had largely elected to stay quiet about the issue, and in exchange, Schumer and his office had completely avoided me. We didn't exchange emails or calls. He'd never even heard me speak—back in 2007 he'd leave press conferences before I was called up. Maybe it was because he was busy. Maybe it was to avoid the press Q&A. Maybe.

Either way, my speech at this 2019 press conference clearly struck Schumer hard. He extended his palm and said, "Do you know why I'm shaking your hand?"

I nodded. "You're Jessica's father."

"Did you know her at school?"

We hadn't been close, but I'd seen on Facebook that she'd just had a baby. I congratulated him on being a new grandfather and he smiled, saying he'd pass along a hello from me. Then he disappeared into the crowd as the presser ended and the gathering dispersed. I heard another advocate chuckling behind me. I turned around and she gave me a mischievous smile. "Seems like you scared him."

AS SOON AS THE post-presser chatter began, it was my turn to dive across the podium, this time to catch the very in-demand Jon Stewart for a photo. We were quickly interrupted by his adoring public—the press pool—so I moved on quickly. To my great disappointment, the room was so hot that I look shiny in all the pictures. My biggest speech ever, and I look haggard in every shot. How does Nancy Pelosi do it?

Before leaving, I asked one of the teacher's union reps to reintroduce me to Rep. Carolyn Maloney, the lead sponsor of every round of Zadroga legislation including, of course, the VCF renewal we were there to introduce. It was her office that had invited me to speak, and not for the first time. Once, at a press conference back in 2007, she'd patted me on the back after my speech and said, "Whoa, do you need a job?" She didn't recognize me in 2019 but, again, told me I should go into politics. My most consistent and most forgetful cheerleader.

As the room cleared out, I left to join some of the advocates for a drink across the street but noticed the blue shirts of the FealGood Foundation moving into a room next door. Nobody said anything about it as they bid me adieu, so I assumed it was nothing—that they were gathering in a room for logistical reasons. Maybe it was where they had left their coats. Maybe they were gathering for one of their famous non-smiling group shots. At a nearby bar a couple of hours later, I learned that they were moving into that room for a reception. Senator Gillibrand had organized a meet and greet for the FealGood Foundation advocates who had come down for the presser. The fact that I wasn't invited, especially as one of the speakers, rubbed me the wrong way. I'd come prepared to butt in, but I was rusty. I didn't remember that, in Washington, you don't wait for invitations. When somebody accidentally tells you what's happening, you just walk into the room and play dumb if people seem irritated to see you there. If you're at the bar across the street, you come back.

The party, by the way, included visits from representatives who had not been at the press conference itself, and I later found out that our recently coronated congressional millennial queen, Rep. Alexandria Ocasio-Cortez, had been among them. That was a bummer. I knew the responders wouldn't be that interested in meeting her because I'd heard them quote conspiracy theories about her, but I very much was. Not just because I admired her very ballsy ascent into the House, but because she was and is open about the challenges of being a young woman in political spaces dominated by men and older people. I wanted to see her operate in that room. Instead I wound up at the table next to a fallen Trump official in a Capitol Hill hotel bar. Washington is a weird place.

I WAS HAPPY TO return to LA later that week and get back to the unpaid, unnoticed voter outreach work I'd been doing. Mostly, I was happy to get away from the FOMO-driven angst that envelops my life whenever I've been in DC for a day too long. Other people experience that in Hollywood,

270 SOME KIDS LEFT BEHIND

but for me DC is Ground Zero for the feeling that everybody is hanging out without you.

In April it was a voting-project-related obligation that brought me back east. I hopped on a plane to New York, then spent several days commuting to a dusty airport hotel near LaGuardia Airport to run a voting workshop for teenagers. The route involved taking a train to a train to a bus, and I was deathly sick with a cold, but the kids were bright, adorable, and motivated. Every day there was pizza and the giddy excitement of one hundred teenagers who are just about to see New York City for the first time. While I was taking the excessively long train ride home on the final day of the workshop, our partners at 9/11 Environmental Action called me to see if I could extend my trip a bit for a forum they were arranging at the Manhattan borough president's office. I said I could.

I was still unemployed, so it was with some relief that I learned that Barasch McGarry's job offer was still open. This time I began asking around in earnest about whether there was any way I could work with them without compromising my contract with 9/11 EA and NIOSH. NIOSH's position, when it was finally elucidated to me, had turned out to be much like their position on my lobbying: I could not do it. Taking the job with Barasch would terminate my contract with them and leave me to fundraise on my own. There was a chance StuyHealth would wind up effectively a subsidiary of Barasch McGarry instead of a public interest organization. At this point, however, I needed the money, and Barasch McGarry was the only VCF firm I knew of putting financial resources and boots on the ground in the renewal effort. They had even hired John Feal, and their lead partner said to me, "Look, we know you want to do this advocacy work, but you have to make a living too." I did know. I just wasn't sure how to manage the clear frustration from the other advocates, my teammates, about my potential relationship with the firm. And then there was managing the relationship with Barasch McGarry itself. The lead partner was famous for making generous donations, then threatening to pull money if the organization's leaders, all of whom were employed full-time under their own nonprofit contracts or by unions, didn't act in a way that aligned with his business needs. I felt like I was caught in a proxy war between a law firm seeking to take advantage of my credibility and advocates threatening to remove that credibility from me if I fought to make a living.

Beyond the outreach contract with NIOSH, I had one other concern as well. Long before the press event in February, I'd asked one of the lead political organizers in the 9/11 health community for his thoughts on how a relationship with Barasch McGarry might complicate my ability to do advocacy work around the Zadroga renewal legislation. He'd been a constant presence in the advocacy scene and ran a c4 financed primarily by unions. In his previous life as a congressional staffer he'd basically written the Zadroga Act, but it meant that along with his voracious advocacy, he could be defensive when it came to its flaws. For years he had been organizing and coordinating the community's political advocacy efforts, and though he was a brilliant tactician he was famously gruff in manner. He said of my potential relationship with Barasch, "It would probably be fine. I mean, I wouldn't use you to testify or anything. But I wouldn't use you for that anyway." I couldn't tell if that was a good or bad answer.

A few months later, in April, as I sat at my parents' kitchen counter, I got a call from the same organizer. "I wanted to see if you'd be available on June 11."

I said, "Sure. For what?"

"Well, it's a secret for now, but we want you to testify at the House Judiciary hearing for the VCF bill." He rushed to add, "But nothing is settled, so no promises. You'd have to get there the night before. Not the morning of, okay?"

As if I'd travel from the West Coast the morning of a hearing. As if I was that kind of big shot.

I said I would definitely be available. I would make myself available by any means necessary. My mouth was probably agape for an hour. My second thought? *Thank God I hadn't committed to anything with the law firm.*

THERE WERE A LOT of reasons that being invited to testify was exciting. It was a chance to tell a part of the survivor story that wasn't well known or understood on the Hill—one in which the government's responsibility for illnesses and injuries is easy to identify. On a more personal level, however, that call also gave my year a mission.

I had known I'd be tangentially involved in the renewal effort, as I always am, but I'd assumed my involvement would be at the whim of a telephone chain that didn't always reach me. My ability to discern the important dates and times to be in DC had, in the past, been heavily reliant on my being party to the right gossip. Now I was finally going to be on the mailing list.

That April, as I entered my sixth month of unemployment, I was less sure than ever about my life's larger direction. I had quit my job to protect my reputation but had not successfully developed an alternative career in entertainment and was beset by a creeping worry that, whatever I did find, I was always going to be an afterthought to people with more important lives and work. My work with StuyHealth has, in the past, been a way of combatting that feeling of inadequacy and insecurity, which is an integral part of the experience of working in Hollywood, but with StuyHealth's funding constantly under threat and my discussions with the law firm complicating my relationships with the other advocates, the anxiety of having no direction began to pull at me on both fronts. Being invited into the belly of the beast to testify, even though I knew there'd still be moments of insecurity, moments of being treated as an afterthought, gave me a reason to look forward to the fight.

With that said, participating in a hearing is a lot more work than it looks like on TV. You don't just slap on a blazer, visit Nancy Pelosi's makeup artist, and get handed a paper to read. First of all, you do your own makeup (and you generally do it wrong because TV and real life offer two very different lighting scenarios). Second of all, when the issue is something an entire community has been working on, everybody wants a piece of your five minutes at the mic. I had to cut Kimberly off when she began sending me testimony line edits via email at fifteen-minute intervals. Then she called me while I was walking down the street with, yes, more line edits. The lead advocate who'd invited me gave me helpful notes on content and delivery but, like Kimberly, caught me only while I was walking down the street. Michael Barasch, the partner at Barasch McGarry who'd been doggedly pursuing me for the job, invited me to discuss a potential post-hearing arrangement and then, mid-meeting, had me recite my testimony for him. He then offered an unsolicited review of my performance.

People had contradictory notes: they wanted to shift the length and focus, they wanted certain facts about the rest of the community mentioned and others erased, and they wanted all of this before I even got the official call to testify from Chairman Nadler's Judiciary Committee staff. When I did get the call, which was just a couple of weeks out, long after I'd finished a draft of the testimony, purchased plane tickets on my own dime, and made housing arrangements, they told me that they hadn't finalized the list of witnesses and were calling simply to gauge my interest. They, too, caught me on the go—I took the call standing at a bench in a Cedars-Sinai hospital parking lot, unsure if I wanted to collapse with exhaustion or burst out laughing. That conversation then launched a flurry of emails and calls—I was desperate to make sure that their exploratory phone call was a formality and that my inclusion in the hearing wasn't up in the air. I was assured by various advocates, who made informal calls to Nadler's staff, that the chairman himself was insisting on my inclusion—that I was definitely going to be on the final list.

Given all of the hubbub and back and forth, by the time I arrived in DC for the big day, I felt like I'd already done the hard part.

AS PROMISED, I FLEW in the day before the hearing. On the morning of June 11 I met a staffer in Nadler's office and was ushered into a waiting room in the maze of the Judiciary Committee's suite. There I saw a group of responders I knew, including Detective Lou Alvarez, who had looked pretty wan back in February and was looking sicker still as he went over his notes. He was only fifty-three years old, heading into his sixty-ninth round of chemo the next day. One of the other responders was tending to a wheelchair meant for him, which he only hesitantly agreed to use and barely fit through the narrow hallways of the committee offices.[270] On the other side of the table was Dr. Jacqueline Moline, the director of the Northwell Health Queens World Trade Center Health Program and a longtime doctor and researcher with the responder program.[271] We'd been on the panel together at that 2018 UFT forum and frequently ran into each other at events. She was seated next to Rupa Bhattacharyya, the special master of the VCF, who had instituted the policy changes that made it easier for survivors to apply. Rupa gave me a comforting smile as I took my seat. John Feal and Jon Stewart were huddled in the far corner discussing whether or not Stewart would give prepared remarks or speak off the cuff. Just before we left to go into the committee chambers, Feal pushed a FealGood Foundation commemorative coin in my direction and smiled. I said my usual refrain, "This is nice, but where's my FealGood Foundation polo shirt?" I'd been bugging him about that for months. He smiled and, as always, asked me for my size. I knew I'd never get the shirt.

A photographer in a FealGood Foundation polo weaved in and out of the chaos as the team awkwardly turned Lou's wheelchair around in the room's narrow entryway. Staffers and elected officials came in and out to offer instructions or to shake hands. Finally, we were ushered down a narrow hallway and through a door that led into the Judiciary Committee hearing chambers. That is, oddly, where my nerves dissipated.

IT MAY BE A cliché that people talk about at protests and in activist corners of the internet, but you rarely get a chance to directly speak truth to power, to find yourself in a room where the people in charge are sitting in front of you waiting for you to speak. I found it intoxicating, the exact opposite of terrifying. As we sat in the audience for the first round of panelists, the two lead sponsors of the House bill, Rupa Bhattacharyya took my hand supportively. Then, as we walked to the witness table, found our name tags, and took a seat, Dr. Moline gave me a comforting pat on the shoulder. As kind as these gestures were, I think they were more for them than for me. I suffer from imposter syndrome almost everywhere—I always have a voice in the back of my head reminding me that I'm not really an expert and people don't really think I belong here. On that day I was surprised to find that I heard nothing of the sort, no internal monologue at all as I sat down for the chair's opening remarks. I settled into my seat, sorted my notes in front of me, and the only thing I said to myself was, *This feels right.* For once, I had no trouble accessing my inner Kara.

That's not to say that I didn't feel some familiar tinges of stress as the witnesses before me began their testimony. Everybody had been told they had five minutes, and I'd carefully cut my comments down to come in just under. Then, just before we began, Dr. Moline and I had a rushed discussion about who to thank at the top of our testimony and how to address them. The results were unwieldy. The hearing was in front of a Judiciary subcommittee, the Subcommittee on the Constitution, Civil Rights, and Civil Liberties chaired by Rep. Steve Cohen of Tennessee, but Chairman Nadler, the full committee's chair, was overseeing the hearing anyway. We debated whether to thank Nadler (yes), Cohen (yes), the opposition's ranking members (maybe), and in what order. I was, as a result, incredibly worried that my thank-yous would eat up too much of my time. It was a relief when I learned that nothing would happen if they did—everybody was going over their allotted time. I wound up being the only person who didn't.

As Dr. Moline finished up just before me, I calmly straightened my

papers. I listened distractedly to Chairman Nadler's introduction as I
rehearsed the intros Dr. Moline and I had decided on. I don't remember
the details, but I remember thinking that I sounded a lot more impressive
in that bio than I'd ever sounded in my own estimation. I also caught a
clever sleight of hand where, after listing all of my StuyHealth-related
accomplishments, Chairman Nadler ended his introduction with, "She
is here testifying in her personal capacity." That was to appease NIOSH,
which had, of course, told me I couldn't testify. Nadler's office had been
exasperated by their interference, though they were accustomed to bizarre
and confusing federal legal demands and the workarounds those sometimes
require. Kimberly had finally brokered a compromise after, similar to our
exchange in February, I'd told her, "I'd rather quit this contract than not
testify," and she'd told me, "I'd rather you get to do both."

When I got the cue, I flipped on my microphone and bumbled through
my thank-yous, forgetting most of the committee members' names and
titles because every single one of them was a mouthful.

"My name is Lila Nordstrom. On September 11 I was a seventeen-year-old student at Stuyvesant, a public high school just three blocks
from the World Trade Center."[272]

I began my comments reading from a paper, but I'd read my testimony
so many times, ushered it through so many edits, that I had whole sections
memorized. Some were passages I'd stolen from rushed press conference
speeches, condensed but familiar.

"On the morning of 9/11 I was in a class with windows looking south.
My classmates and I saw planes hit the Twin Towers, dozens of people
jumping to their deaths, and thousands of evacuees streaming out of the
area. Then the first tower fell, and a dust cloud started to rush toward us,
and suddenly we couldn't see anything."[273]

I didn't feel nervous, but when I checked the C-SPAN feed later my
hands were shaking, so I must have had some anxious energy coursing
through me. Whatever my hands were doing, my mental focus was

exceptional. I was on. I felt the pressure of the moment, but for once I was able to view it as an opportunity, not a potential disappointment or failure, not a cause for embarrassment, nothing like what my anxiety usually imposes. My whole adult life, I'd been angling for the chance to have that exact moment, to have my classmates' and my experience finally put on the record. As students, we'd been largely overlooked by the city's two 9/11 museums, largely overlooked by the media's account of 9/11, even overlooked by our own school alumni because anybody who wasn't there in 2001 and 2002 had immense difficulty imagining what we'd dealt with just to go to school. This was a chance to correct that record.

"After EPA Administrator Christine Todd Whitman assured New Yorkers that the air downtown was 'safe to breathe,' government officials decided to send us back. Stuyvesant returned on October 9, less than a month after the attacks."[274]

I quickly went over the government's grossest acts of negligence. "The smell of smoke was suffocating, and despite assurances from officials, very little was done to prepare the school for students. No hazmat team got called in. The filters in our ventilation system weren't replaced until January, the WTC dust sitting in our air vents wasn't removed until the following summer, and the auditorium's contaminated upholstery wasn't fully replaced until 2014, more than ten years later."[275]

At that point I gestured to a display, two images that Congressman Nadler's office had printed and carted into the room. One was a photo of a news article from 2014. I'd been told I could bring a visual aid, but when I suggested a few photos, other advocates told me to bring only two and only those I could dramatically gesture to during my testimony. I forgot to point to the first one, a slightly blurred image of students entering Stuyvesant in 2001 in front of the garbage barge taken by my good friend Ethan Moses. The second, a clipping of an online news article about the Stuyvesant theater's reupholstery in 2014, was also projected on a large screen behind me. It wasn't quite the exciting smoking-gun moment I'd planned, but it was effective enough as it hovered there, reminding the members of the committee how long we'd sat in these dangers.

I was given a tall order in my testimony. Three responders and a responder's widow went right on the heels of my remarks, and all testified about different aspects of the responder experience. I, by contrast, was the only community representative there. Though I was telling the student story, I had to work in many other aspects of the 9/11 community experience as well, to remember I was speaking for over three hundred thousand of the event's most voiceless victims.[276] That gave me a lot of ground to cover. I did not personally have to clean up any contaminated spaces without guidance or safety gear, but members of the community did, so I mentioned the "dangerously inadequate guidance"[277] they were given. In my notes the word "dangerously" was underlined so I'd remember to stress it.

I ended the testimony with a reminder of my youth. "The youngest 9/11 survivors have to live with the results of these exposures for another seventy or eighty years. Cancer does not respect arbitrary funding deadlines. If the VCF is allowed to reduce payouts and expire, a resource meant to ease our suffering is going to become yet another symbol of how we were sacrificed by a government that thought a quick return to normalcy after a tragic event was more important than the health and safety of the children who lived through it."[278]

I was the first of the 9/11 victims to speak, meaning mine was the first story of trauma that people in the room heard that day. They would, of course, hear many more, but the student story had the distinction of being the only one that they had never actually heard before. For some, it was the first time they'd heard about kids being impacted at all.

As with most hearings, there were very few members of Congress sitting in the committee room during my remarks. Those absences are pretty normal, although Jon Stewart would make a very theatrical point about them during his later testimony, a brilliant move that the media narrative really seized on. Taken as a whole, the panel of victims I kicked off was incredibly impactful and, at times, hard to listen to—the witness next to me, Anesta Maria St. Rose Henry, whose first responder husband, Candidus Henry, had died two weeks prior of brain cancer at age fifty-two,[279] broke down in tears during her remarks. I wasn't expecting her sudden display of emotion and wasn't sure how to react in such a formal environmental, so I rubbed her back lightly as her children behind us encouraged her to go on.

Still, it was, as planned, Jon Stewart's remarks on the heels of Detective Lou Alvarez's dramatic appearance that caused the hearing to go viral. Detective Alvarez reminded the panel, "You made me come down here the day before my sixty-ninth round of chemo, and I'm going to make sure that you never forget to take care of the 9/11 responders."[280]

The room, filled with a sea of blue FealGood Foundation polo shirts, had given him a standing ovation—I nearly kneecapped the person behind me as I pushed my heavy chair back in time to stand. Stewart worked off of the room's heavy, emotional energy and drove home the obvious cruelty of making us perform at this hearing in the first place. He swept in, indignant, having decided (with John Feal's encouragement) to abandon his written remarks and speak off the cuff. He did so brilliantly.

"I want to thank Mr. Collins and Mr. Nadler for putting this together. But, as I sit here today," he began, "I can't help but think what an incredible metaphor this room is for the entire process that getting health care and benefits for 9/11 first responders has come to."

He continued. "Behind me: a filled room of 9/11 first responders. And in front of me: a nearly empty Congress. Sick and dying, they brought themselves down here to speak—to no one."[281]

The room behind him, packed with responders and survivors, egged him on. He was not his usual slyly comic self, and he was not interested in playing the propriety game.

"I'm sorry if I sound angry and undiplomatic, but I'm angry—and you should be too; and they're all angry as well. And they have every justification to be that way. There is not a person here, there is not an empty chair on that stage that didn't tweet out, 'Never forget' the heroes of 9/11; never forget their bravery; never forget what they did, what they gave to this country."[282]

I don't think there was a point at which I knew his speech would go viral. I assumed the entire affair would happen under the radar, as these things usually do, but there was one line in the middle that struck me. A line that felt so apt that I echoed it just a few weeks later on the eve of the House vote. He said, "Your indifference cost these men and women their most valuable commodity: time. It's the one thing they're running out of." All of us on that panel were fighting for different kinds of time, and Congress kept wasting what, for us, was an especially limited resource.

The final moments of Stewart's speech were repeated on every news network that night, referencing the amount of time it took for the first of the responders to answer the call on 9/11. "They responded in five seconds. They did their jobs with courage, grace, tenacity, humility. Eighteen years later—do yours!"[283] Americans ate it up.

UNSURPRISINGLY, CONSIDERING STEWART'S POWER-HOUSE remarks and Lou Alvarez's heart-wrenching appeals, the rest of us didn't make it into any coverage. A lot of my Facebook friends posted about the hearing without noting (or, frankly, knowing) that I was there. There was, however, a larger story that was only evident if you watched the entire hearing.

After Stewart spoke the hearing didn't end. It droned on for another hour as committee members made comments or asked questions. In that second hour, before we had a chance to see how the media would run with the story, I found myself emerging as the star witness. In their queries and comments, members of Congress kept bringing it back to me.

Chairman Nadler began the questioning with a real zinger. After describing the actions of the EPA that assured New Yorkers the air was safe to breathe, he turned to me and asked, "As a matter of moral responsibility, do you agree that Congress, as representatives of the American people, should help to give some measure of compensation to the victims for the harms they have suffered that were exacerbated by the government's own actions at the time?"[284]

"I think they absolutely should," I answered. "I'm sitting before you as someone who was present on 9/11, but I was not caught in the dust cloud. There is no reason that my respiratory health, or my gastrointestinal health . . . should have been impacted by the events of 9/11. I only have these conditions because I was sent back, and I was sent back because the federal government assured New Yorkers that the air downtown was safe to breathe."[285]

A few minutes later Rep. Jamie Raskin of Maryland turned to me. "Ms. Nordstrom, I want to ask you a question. Your story is very poignant to me. You are describing what happened to schoolchildren who were sent back to the neighborhood when it was no longer safe. And now you describe how many of your classmates are coming down with asthma and cancer and fatal diseases. And you have already lost some of them in your—I think you described being at your twentieth reunion? Is that right?"[286]

He'd aged me up. "Not even my twentieth reunion," I replied.

He continued. "How does America or how does the city keep track of people in your situation? Who reached out to you? I assume the fire departments have a way of communicating with people, but who was keeping track of people in your situation?"[287]

The simple answer would have been that nobody reached out. That I had volunteered myself to be that person. What I said was, "That has been incredibly challenging. And one of the reasons that this fund closing when it does will really be harmful for us is that a lot of people in my situation are not aware that they qualify for these services."[288] I talked about the challenges of living out of state. I talked about the challenges of reaching people who never lived in the area to begin with. I ended with, "We are still doing the work of reaching out to them now."[289]

Soon after, Rep. Madeleine Dean of Pennsylvania came to me. "Ms. Nordstrom, I think your testimony is particularly compelling. Can you describe more about what notices you were given, even as young students, or your parents were given or your teachers were given about the status of the health in your school?"[290]

I thought immediately of the water fountains. "Once we were already back at the school we received a number of cryptic warnings. We started to get notes home that said don't drink out of the water fountain, and we were suddenly not allowed to leave the building for lunch, which was a privilege that we had enjoyed before that. And, for some reason, it was supposed to be okay that we walked to and from the subway in that same air, but apparently eating lunch was not going to be safe."

I went on to talk about how little we could do about the situation as children. "As soon as we were back, a sort of contentious discussion broke out about whether we should be there or not. But, you know, we didn't really have any agency in that discussion. That was obviously a discussion that was happening between government officials, parents, and teachers at the school."

I described how the Parents' Association had later discovered things weren't as safe as they seemed. I made my most serious charge at the government yet, stressing that it was clear that we should have never been there but that we never received that information at a point where we could have acted on it.

"Certainly," I told her, "if the government officials charged with our care had been honest about the situation, I think it would have been appropriate to remove us from the premises."

She responded with, "It sounds like malpractice to me." I almost smiled at her in thanks for saying it, blowing my aggrieved victim scowl (I'd been warned many times and said it myself: hearings are 50 percent theater).

But it *was* malpractice, and it was nice to hear somebody from behind a government dais, somebody who wasn't a New Yorker herself and therefore personally tied to the situation, say it on the record.

These questions were not the usual, long-winded semi-rhetorical questions responders always get about whether 9/11 was hard (of course it was) or whether they feel pride in their work (of course they do). In my case the committee wanted to know more about how students had been lied to, mistreated, and left in danger by a government eager to get things back to normal. They needed to know because nobody had told them this information before, at least not in a context in which they'd had to listen. My story was the one that made them think about their own districts and how they'd want the people in that district to be treated after a major catastrophe. I seized on the chance to give information I hadn't had time to include in my original testimony. After the questions, I felt like I'd hit most of what I came there to say.

LATER, SEVERAL PEOPLE, INCLUDING some committee members, staffers, and a few general-purpose Hill rats, told me that though the Stewart narrative was dominant in the coverage, it was my testimony that lit a fire under everybody in the room. I absolutely felt that. Rep. Sheila Jackson Lee came up to me afterward as we all milled about in the room and told me they should make sure to invite me back for the Senate hearings (though there didn't turn out to be any). I took that as a sign that I'd done something right.

Post-hearing, the atmosphere in the room became oddly festive. I chatted with a few other committee members, soliciting stories from Chairman Nadler about his days at Stuyvesant High School with infamous conservative political operative Dick Morris and longtime New York State assemblyman Dick Gottfried. He'd seemed tired and exasperated during the hearing, but in telling those old stories he came alive. Kara, who was working on the Hill and had ducked out of her office to watch the end of the questioning, snapped some photos of the moment his face lit up. Another advocate asked, "What on earth did you say to him?"

After the room began to empty out and the interest in group photos began to wane, John Feal announced, as if we were a high school class visiting the Capitol, that it was lunchtime and we'd meet back in an hour. Something I overheard, however, made clear he and Stewart had other things planned. Michael Barasch waved me over and whispered, "Just follow us," to me. Not wanting to relive my February disappointment at missing the post-presser reception, I did. I kept my gaze on my phone so that nobody would be able to give me questioning looks or catch my attention to tell me to buzz off. (In retrospect it shocks me that, even after testifying, I instinctively felt I might not be important enough for the follow-up visits. That memory of 2015 was still lodged somewhere deep.) Eyes on my phone, I followed the group straight into the Rayburn Room in the Capitol, an ornate conference room, where I asked Jon Stewart if he'd be willing to do an outreach video geared to students and he said yes. Then I followed them straight into Nancy Pelosi's office, where we met the Speaker and took photos on the Speaker's balcony.

After that photo op, I stopped pretending to follow and started to do it openly. We next marched as a group to a rotunda that many Capitol Hill reporters use for their live shots and did the press rounds. I got sent to do some of the digital news interviews, and because of that I didn't make it into the live shot for the main appearance they were there to do—an interview with Shep Smith on Fox News. What I did instead was stand opposite them, just next to the camera, and take photos of them with their phones. I did it so I could catch the group members' eyes if need be. When Jon Stewart began to speak, I listened carefully and stared directly at him as he, perhaps accidentally, set himself up to mention the community.

One of the bizarre things about Stewart as an advocate was that he never mentioned the community side of the 9/11 health issue. He even lived in the community after 9/11, breathing in the same toxic air as the rest of us, but I could never tell if he just didn't know there was a health crisis there too or wasn't interested. He'd had a Schumer-like avoidance of acknowledging our piece of the puzzle, and even when he did mention his own experience living down there, it was always in service of a point about how responders helped his community heal.

When I made eye contact with him that day, though, fresh off that hearing where he'd listened to me answer rounds of questions and heard so much of the community story in depth, he suddenly, as if by magic, remembered 9/11's students. That caused him to mention the community. Suddenly he was talking about how we'd been down there with responders and framed us as worthy recipients of the Zadroga services, the first time I'd ever heard him do that, and on Fox News no less. I quietly took full credit for it, for my impeccably timed glare. When the shot was over and one of the advocates bemoaned that I hadn't made it into the shot, I said to myself, *Yes, I did.*

Stewart's comment did me an additional favor the next day too. I didn't get to do much in the way of media after the hearing itself—I got invited to do CNN's Don Lemon that night but they later disinvited me, telling me they'd found a responder instead, as if I'd obviously understand that of course any responder (it was not even one who'd testified!) was a better guest than I was. Aside from those live shots, the only press I did in the aftermath of the hearing was actually a Fox News interview with Shep Smith, the very same man who'd heard Stewart's mention. I credit that comment for creating a space for me somewhere on a national news network.

I had mixed feelings about the fact that Fox News was the only place I was able to tell the community story, of course. I am well aware of its role in the rise of Trumpism and its willingness to create space for the kinds of dangerous policy and thought that work against my broader health policy goals, not to mention my most basic social justice priorities. This wasn't the first time they had shown interest, either. My first big, live-via-satellite interview had also been with Fox News, back in 2011. Kimberly Guilfoyle spoke to me in what was my first national interview about the survivor community and students specifically. It was in her pre-Trump family days, back when she was mostly famous for her marriage with California governor Gavin Newsom. I did the interview at Fox News's LA studios on my way to Santa Monica, where I was late for my production assistant gig on some commercial for Kmart.

Fox News famously loves a salacious story about government incompetence, which is probably why they've been willing to report on nonresponders where other networks have not, but I still found their lone interest in our cause bizarre. Certainly, in an era of biased cable news networks, it was not the network known for dog whistles and conspiracy-laden infotainment that I thought would be interested in a cause that's essentially about community justice. Of course, they weren't exactly inviting Chinatown or Lower East Side residents, who make up a large part of our survivor cohort, on air to discuss the issue. But the fact that survivor community members never got mentioned once on CNN or MSNBC and instead found our only national press opportunities at Fox News was head-scratching. Conservatives whom I don't agree with on almost anything are considerably more likely than my progressive friends to know that my community was put in danger after 9/11, and that's weird.

The Fox interview was on the day following the hearing at their DC bureau in an office building not far from the Hill. They sent a car to pick me up, which I loaded my suitcase into, planning to go straight to the train station as soon as the interview was over. The waiting room was empty save one other commentator, an expert in Middle Eastern politics. We watched Fox's coverage of an incredibly bizarre Trump press conference as we waited, both unsure of whether we were in safe enough company to acknowledge that a trick of light was making it look like Trump was bald. Finally, he commented on how funny it was that nobody was doing anything about the Trump hair issue and I agreed, flushed with relief.

After a brief conversation with Shep Smith filmed from a small, windowless chamber, I headed straight to the train, still caked in Fox News makeup and hairspray. Barasch McGarry had offered to buy me a ticket on the Acela so that I didn't have to sweat it out on the bus for five hours, an opportunity for which I was grateful as I tried to take off some of the layers of blush and concealer that had been plastered onto my face for my two minutes of camera time. I'd done a number of TV interviews by that point, but Fox News remains the only place where they've asked, as a matter of course, if I want fake lashes. (I declined and told them to make me look natural, but "natural" at Fox is its own animal.) Later John Feal told me I would have looked better without all that makeup. As if Fox News gives women that choice. As if society does.

I flew back to LA a few days later, still reeling from the excitement of the hearing, but found myself back on a plane only a couple of weeks after, having been again invited by Rep. Carolyn Maloney's office to speak at the press conference that would be held just before the House vote on the Zadroga renewal. Unlike past pressers, this one would feature Nancy Pelosi herself. Though I'd met her, now twice, I'd never had to speak in front of her. That seemed like a dramatically different ask. What do you say when the media isn't going to remember you but the Speaker of the House might?

The day of the vote I was taken over to the Speaker's office by Representative Maloney's staff. I nervously eyed a bowl of chocolates as other speakers, staffers, and politicians arrived. We milled. When Pelosi burst in, shaking the room awake, we all jumped to attention. She shook our hands, then had a conversation about strategy with Jon Stewart, whose celebrity gave him the entrée to ask a lot of direct questions that the rest of us couldn't. On the way to the presser I just happened to be walking next to Rep. Peter King, the lead Republican sponsor of the Zadroga Act, and he casually complimented me on my performance at the hearing, saying, "Interesting story you told about the students. I'd never heard about that before."

If he'd never heard it, it was because he'd never listened. He'd been in Congress since 1993 and the lead Republican on this issue for years, and yet somehow I'd been the first person to get him to truly listen to the student survivor story in all that time. Either I'd done something right or we'd all done something wrong. Hard to know.

There were some new faces in the crowd as we gathered. Detective Alvarez had just died—I'd been out of town for his deservedly large and highly publicized funeral procession, which took place only a few weeks after the hearing. His family had been invited to speak on his behalf and had taken over the responsibility of carrying his message forward with great earnestness. As soon as we walked en masse into a large room filled with reporters and members of Congress, his sister, Aida, turned to me and said, "Do you think I can do my speech in Spanish?" I told her she should do whatever she needed to.

We gathered behind the podium and waited as umpteen members of Congress spoke; then, one by one, we were invited up. Aida delivered fantastic remarks, partly in Spanish but her point was clear to all of us. I was last, as usual, but thinking back on Stewart's remarks at the hearing and Representative King's comment on the way to the room, I decided that, given the captive audience and more importantly the new high-profile addition to my podium posse, I would speak about something a little different. Usually I tell the student story, and I covered some of that, but this time I focused on how long I'd been making the trips down to Washington, how for thirteen years I'd been walking the halls of Congress with the people who were seated behind me. How, for me, this was my entire adult life. I think it was an effective point. It put me on the Speaker's radar, for one, and let the audience of reporters and politicos know their inaction had stolen a piece of my youth, but it also reminded the rest of the advocates that I'd been there with them all along.

After the presser we rushed to the House gallery for the vote. They were voting on a series of national security bills for what felt like hours before they got to ours, but the House members broke into applause as our bill passed. In the following excitement I finally met Rep. Alexandria Ocasio-Cortez, who came up to the balcony to shake our hands. I chatted with her staff briefly, then got lost in the Capitol looking for the rest of the crew. One of the Speaker's staffers found me wandering the halls and directed me to the area where John Feal, Jon Stewart, and a bunch of responders were doing interviews. I naturally made it just in time for Fox, where Feal, with his impeccable sense of drama, teared up, then gave me a big hug on-screen. For the first time, I felt like I had the power to invite myself to be there. That I didn't need to wait for the approval of other advocates to walk into the live shot. Every interview they gave after I arrived included a mention of students, of residents, of the survivor community in general. With my speech that day and the freedom that came from the bill's new momentum, we had effectively rewritten the story to include us.

That Monday I continued my press tour, appearing at a press conference down by the World Trade Center that was focused on pressuring the Senate to schedule a vote. I arrived clad in casual faded pink jeans and a T-shirt, my hair blowing everywhere as I stood in a windy corridor of downtown buildings, trying to remember my talking points. I gesticulated wildly as I exclaimed, "We need to see some commitment from the Senate now. We need to set a date to vote and make sure that this program is protected." I veered back into the talking points I'd debuted in front of Nancy Pelosi as well.

"I myself made my first trip down to Washington to advocate for the needs of 9/11 survivors in 2007. I was twenty-two years old. I went back in 2009 and 2010 to advocate for the passage of the Zadroga Act. I went back five years later to advocate for the renewal. And I'll go back as many times as it takes, but I have spent my entire twenties, and half of my thirties, walking the halls of Congress, telling the story of the scariest day and the scariest year of my life. Telling stories about my personal health issues. About those of my friends. All of this in excruciating details, and on repeat.

These are really hard trips to make. Every trip down there is a reminder that the government used us to make sure that Wall Street was back on its feet instead of taking care of the children that were in the direct line of the attack. Every trip is a reminder that there is a black cloud hanging over my health and my future."[291]

I ended on a plea. "Instead of ending this program, let's end the charade where we go down to Washington and beg Congress to care about us after experiencing a health crisis that the government's own policy helped create."[292] I demanded a vote. As usual, Senator Schumer had left before I got up to speak, but the responders gathered behind me cheered me on supportively as I closed out the event and went back to my spot in the crowd, back to being a random woman in salmon-colored jeans amid a sea of FealGood Foundation polo shirts.

THE SENATE FEIGNED INDIFFERENCE to our pleas, but it seemed like action might be forthcoming. I decided to stay on the East Coast to wait out the Senate vote in upstate New York. While I was there, I got a rushed call asking if I could go on *The Late Show with Stephen Colbert* with a group of responders that night. I was ready to jump into a car that moment, but much to my everlasting disappointment Jon Stewart ended up going on by himself. The idea was to push Senate Majority Leader Mitch McConnell to sit down with responders, and the pressure got so high that he finally did. McConnell promised to schedule a vote, and a couple weeks later we made our way back to DC to watch that vote happen.

The day of the Senate vote, I was, true to form, early, and passed some time chatting with a *Daily News* reporter who'd been shadowing the FealGood Foundation lobbyists for some time and had seen me many times on the Hill. While we talked, the lead advocate, the one who had invited me to testify and had orchestrated our behind-the-scenes strategy, came by. The reporter casually said to him, "I hear Lila is speaking today," and he looked at the reporter and said, "Yeah, she's speaking last, but she's speaking." I still don't know whether he meant that as a putdown (my interpretation at the time) or an expression of frustration (Kimberly's take on it later). Either way, it put me in a sour mood, and even the reporter, who wasn't exactly heaping community mentions into his own stories, looked at me quizzically and conspiratorially, like, *What was that?*

Soon after, the FealGood Foundation guys, who always gathered beforehand to take pictures and get a pep talk from John Feal, made a dramatic entrance, tailed by cameras, high-fiving people as they went. John Feal and Jon Stewart both gave me big hugs. High drama for posterity. Detective Alvarez's family was back and took turns embracing me as well before heading off to the side to do interviews. They were, by now, toughened press experts. We stood around in the hallway as a mass, causing chaos outside Senator Gillibrand's office, with John Feal periodically breaking up the fun in his best middle school teacher/army captain voice to yell at everybody about behaving, then remind everybody they'd get pizza later.

In those final months, I learned a lot about how much work John Feal had done all those years not just in dealing with Congress but in keeping everybody on the FealGood side in line. With so many of his guys coming out of law enforcement and other militantly hierarchical professions, the FealGood team generally responded to his brand of alpha authority, but there were always shenanigans. He didn't sleep so he could enforce a curfew and make sure responders weren't staying out late partying. He would often make announcements reminding people to behave themselves when things got rowdy in the halls of Congress. He'd kick guys out of his squad who weren't disciplined or serious about the cause. By 2019 his teams were mostly responsible, kind, and very dedicated. He'd often remark on how many bad eggs they'd had to move out since 2010, but whatever his methods, and I know they took a lot out of him, his final bunch was definitely a team of good eggs.

John Feal's hands-on management and team-building style also filtered down to me. He wasn't shy about sharing tips. One was to stop using my hands so much when I spoke in front of people. The other was to not worry about wearing makeup on TV, though I think this was because he liked to refuse makeup and was trying to get an army of us together to do it with him. Finally, that I should get married. I'm not sure how that was related to the other two, but I figured that since he hadn't gotten me a FealGood polo shirt, despite my many requests, I didn't have to listen to him.

The rest of my own team, the other survivor advocates, who had once again bowed to the optics and been notably and intentionally absent from a lot of the early events, finally got a chance to come down for the Senate vote. It was exciting considering they'd been, over the years, pretty directly uninvited from every other aspect of the lobbying process (usually followed by them being criticized for not showing up, but alas, such is life). Kimberly was there, and she and I walked into the Senate Chambers together, taking a seat next to Caryn Pfeifer, the widow of Ray Pfeifer. Ray had been a fire-fighter and passionate responder advocate—he was one of the guys who had appeared on the *Daily Show* back in 2010 and came, wheelchair-bound and ailing, to outreach and advocacy events until soon before his death in 2017. He was always smiling, and his family now manages a foundation in his name that helps sick firefighters cover necessary expenses. His wife watched in nervous anticipation, vocalizing her need for a cigarette several times.

Before the House vote, the Zadroga Act's title had been amended to include Ray's and Detective Alvarez's names. The full title now read "Never Forget the Heroes: James Zadroga, Ray Pfeifer, and Luis Alvarez Permanent Authorization of the September 11th Victim Compensation Fund Act." It was unwieldy to be sure, and generally hilarious to watch anybody try to say, but it was a nice tribute to the work Ray and Lou had done.

We were seated in the gallery during remarks in opposition to the VCF renewal from the two senators preventing a unanimous consent vote, Sen. Rand Paul and Sen. Mike Lee (the very same guy whom we'd all taken that creepy meeting with in 2015 where he asked for gory details of the rescue).

We waited, and waited, then scoured the Senate floor as the vote finally came up and the members slowly appeared. Sen. Gillibrand and Senator Cory Gardner of Colorado, the bill's GOP sponsor, paced the clerk's desk, keeping an eye on everybody. Early in was Sen. Amy Klobuchar, who cast a yes vote. We felt good when we saw GOP Sen. Joni Ernst cast her yes vote early, assuming this meant the GOP wasn't going to be unified in opposition. Ernst then chatted with Senator Gillibrand for a while—we speculated that this was because Ernst is from Iowa, the first state up in the 2020 primaries, and Gillibrand was running for president. Sen. Cory Booker, ever the fan of the cool-guy entrance, showed up and fist-bumped the pages as he cast his vote. Sen. Kamala Harris, like Gillibrand and Klobuchar a presidential hopeful, strolled in. She was still my junior senator from California at the time, not yet a historic vice president, and though she looks so tall on television and when she's eviscerating people in committee, she was petite in person, standing slightly below the eyelines of the gathering men in suits. She cast her yes vote. Not petite? Sen. Dianne Feinstein, my other California senator, who, probably because she was the oldest member of the senate, I assumed was going to be tiny. She's actually quite tall, which made it especially easy to find her as she, hilariously, held on to her pocketbook in a manner that suggested she was worried about pickpockets on the Senate floor. She cast her yes vote. At the very last moment, the controversial conservative Sen. Ted Cruz burst into the room and proudly cast a yes vote too. In a contentious session in which the Senate was being criticized as the place legislation goes to die, senators on both sides of the aisle looked excited just to have something meaningful to do. When the final count came, the vote was 98–2. We cheered, then got yelled at by the sergeant at arms and threatened with arrest (nobody is supposed to make noise in the Senate gallery; it's all very polite and decorum-obsessed). We didn't care, though. We felt invincible.

After the vote we rushed into a nearby press room and one by one made remarks commenting on how relieved we were and how we hoped the president would sign the bill without trouble. Somebody kept leaning on the light switch, so periodically we'd all find ourselves suddenly thrust into the dark. We'd recover, and then it would happen again.

As the last speaker in a hot room that nobody was interested staying in much longer, I knew I'd probably not make it into any coverage, so I focused on saying something useful to my work, something we could use on StuyHealth's social media as part of our own survivor outreach efforts. I decided to speak about how we rarely see ourselves reflected in coverage and said, in no uncertain terms, repeating it as often as I could, "This program is for you, too."

THE RESPONDERS INVITED ME to their dinner outside DC, but I wanted to spend the evening with my personal support crew. Kara and I went out to dinner to celebrate that night, and I made plans to get back to New York and finally fly back to LA, where my apartment was in shambles and life was on hold. Then, close to midnight, I got an email from Speaker Pelosi's press staff asking if I was available the following morning to attend a ceremony. The House and Senate sponsors of the bill were holding their own signing ceremony, making the (correct) assumption that they'd never get invited to the White House for the president's signing. (I did ultimately get invited to the White House signing ceremony. I never thought I'd turn down an invite to the White House, but the Trump era was an extraordinary time. I had to say no. In a blatant show of partisanship, the only member of Congress who was invited was Rep. Peter King. When I asked some of my FealGood Foundation friends about it later, most of them simply commented that it had been hot.)

I had no mixed feelings about the House event, which I enthusiastically said yes to. I showed up that morning expecting to find the usual suspects. Instead, it was just me and four union reps.

The reputation of the union reps was always that they were mostly there to take credit for work that other people were on the floor actually doing, though I'm sure most of them used their political connections and leverage to help support the cause. The benefit, however, was that I was the only recognizable advocate at the event. I was the Jon Stewart of that room.

The ceremony was a photo op, mostly organized so that various members of the New York delegation who had supported the legislation could be a part of something. Because of my diminutive height, I got pushed into the front of the huddle. The union reps, with their suits and tall stature, got pushed to the back and hovered behind the scene, floating mops of hair invisible behind the crowd. In the resulting photos, I'm the only advocate visible in a sea of members of Congress. Chuck Schumer jumped in and out to cast a vote, then chuckled about it with everybody. One of the members of Congress went to the same high school as me, and we chatted about our time there and people we knew in common. Then, at the end, holding one of the pens that were used to sign the bill, I took a photo with Rep. Carolyn Maloney and Speaker Pelosi, and as I walked away, the Speaker grabbed my hand and said, "Don't be a stranger."

Moments later, a little starry-eyed, I was released back into my regular life.

CHAPTER 13

THE AMERICAN
DISASTER VICTIM

The rhetoric around 9/11 is always that it was this massive singular event that will never be replicated. That we should #NeverForget it. That it's special.

It's not. Little 9/11s happen constantly. We often create them out of situations that didn't have to be disasters at all.

Unsurprisingly, the people who suffer the most in disasters big and small are often the people with the least agency—kids. Every day in America, millions of children head to school worried that a random act of gun violence could end their lives.[293] Kids in Flint, Michigan, prepare for school without clean water or living with the complicated legacies of having gone years without that resource.[294] Kids in New Orleans, Louisiana, and Houston, Texas, get dressed in homes and neighborhoods still dealing with flood damage or flooding anew.[295] Kids in California wake up in neighborhoods suffused with smoke from acres-wide fires and have to pretend it's like any other day.[296] Kids living in pandemic hot zones or, frankly, anywhere in America in 2020 and 2021, watch their world shrink overnight.[297] The experience of 9/11 may have been on a larger scale than a few of these, an act of mass violence paired with a major health and environmental disaster, but that doesn't mean that these individual crises aren't bad enough on their own. Lives are irrevocably changed by smaller disasters too.

Often the way we process the scale of a disaster isn't really about how big it is, anyway. A lot of big and little 9/11s happen to kids and communities that don't have the coattails of responders or other designated "heroes" to ride or financial resources to throw around or voices the media is willing to seek out. Even with the clarifying effect that the COVID-19 pandemic has had on many Americans, we at most do some hand-wringing in the media. We ask, "What did we do to create this problem?" Then we do nothing.

The ideological and political right would often have you believe that the "nothing" response is because we did nothing in the first place—that problems sometimes just pop up out of thin air, that sometimes people are just unlucky or, more commonly, that the people themselves brought on the problem by moving to a certain neighborhood, sending their kids to a certain school, or simply failing to protect themselves from dangers they could not see. The left, by contrast, would have you believe that our social contract with these people has been broken. That we make reckless policy choices that make acts of mass violence possible, that we sentence unsuspecting people to suffering from inevitable worsening environmental risks by refusing to take action to stop them beforehand. That, sometimes, we create the bad luck that people experience.

Oftentimes, of course, we forget to ask any questions at all, because answering them requires too much work or because a newer, sexier crisis has already emerged on the horizon. Occasionally, when adults fail to take proper stock of the situation, we leave kids to ask what's going on themselves. March for Our Lives, the impressive organization that was formed by student survivors in the aftermath of the school shooting at Marjory Stoneman Douglas High School in Parkland, Florida,[298] is an outgrowth of a system in which adults shirked their duty to think critically about the role they had played in creating a crisis. It shouldn't have been on the kids who were victimized to inquire about the policies that led to their trauma, but somebody had to.

As far as answers to these questions go, I'm partial to the left's point of view. I think we could make choices to slow or stop many of the disasters that destroy lives both here and abroad if we cared to. If we learn anything from the slow-rolling, still simmering COVID-19 crisis, I hope it's this: That preemptive action to save people from suffering is always a good idea. That it's worth a risk to the economy to make sure people are safe. People are our most important asset, not financial indicators. In the aftermath of a crisis, however, I don't think that we should be initially preoccupied with *how* we allowed the crisis to happen. When the damage is done, what we should ask first is, "How can we protect survivors from further harm?"

People rarely mention the unpleasant reality that is living with the long-term consequences of a disaster, but we do see glimmers of it in the news sometimes in reports, for example, about GoFundMe accounts popping up for gunshot victims and cancer patients. (Medical bills account for one third of GoFundMe's business, and crowdfunding platforms have become one of the main ways that American families pay for sudden health expenses.[299]) Substance abuse and suicide rates skyrocket among post-disaster populations, too.[300] Traumatized adults make terrible decisions that traumatize kids further in the name of safety. We think we're addressing the question of how to prevent further harm while asking Stuyvesant students to wear IDs, claiming that is how we will protect them from terrorists. Or asking kids in Parkland to use clear backpacks to protect them from guns.[301] Or watching kids in Flint bathe in donated bottled water.[302]

Unfortunately, wearing IDs doesn't clean the air at Stuyvesant, nor does it make the student body feel safer from terrorism. Clear backpacks in Parkland inflicted their own trauma because they were a visual reminder that something terrifying had happened recently and that nothing would ever be the same. Old gunshot wounds remain painful and problematic,

even when everybody wears clear backpacks and goes through sixteen security checkpoints on the way into school. Bathing in bottled water doesn't
stop Flint's kids from experiencing the effects of having already bathed in
and ingested contaminated water.

We ignore the elephant in the room and make choices that compound
the trauma, but, of course, the trauma is also the problem. It's not just
because giving people all the ingredients for a PTSD diagnosis is a terrible
idea, although obviously it is. Trauma is the problem because trauma in the
American context is expensive. Trauma becomes its own crisis. It evolves
into stress-related heart conditions and substance abuse issues.[303] It becomes
depression.[304] All of that is in addition to the other health woes many of
these populations must navigate. What binds disaster kids and disaster
communities together is more visible on GoFundMe than in the words and
admonitions of the politicians and people who make it their business to
#NeverForget or offer "thoughts and prayers," because trauma cheats us out
of our value: our time, our money, our opportunities, our sanity.

"Preventing further harm" is also not just about addressing one bad
corporate policy or foreign policy or gun policy or environmental policy.
It's about addressing the main thing that puts us disaster kids in a long-term
bind—bad health policy. The absence of basic health care protections in
America, even in the post–Affordable Care Act era, is at the very crux of
what fails to protect survivors meaningfully from further harm.

While we regularly put millions of America's children, as well as their
families and communities, through a series of ceaseless, unnecessary, and
cruel crises, we act like these events have nothing to do with health care.
The thing is, though every disaster is distinct, America breaks its social
contract with the survivors in the same way every time: the same neglect
my classmates and I faced regarding our health needs regularly imperils
thousands of kids in the aftermath of their own scary situations, whether
they be caused by climate change, acts of mass violence, a pandemic, or just
random bad luck. The neglect is about what we don't provide, not what we

don't prevent. It's that we don't have consistent, affordable, and easy access to health care in the aftermath.

So why are we so keen to avoid the elephant in the room—that a major disaster leaves communities in need in ways that are far more holistic and go far beyond addressing the scourge of opaque backpacks and ID-less breastbones? That a structure that could protect us meaningfully from future harm, and is available almost everywhere else in the developed world,[305] is so startlingly absent in our system? In the late 2000s I wrote in *The Guardian*:

> 'Small government'-style social policy has not served 9/11 victims well. Community groups have had to fight tooth and nail for often meager funding that comes in one-time bursts. There are still no medical monitoring and few treatment programs available to the thousands of people who were exposed to the toxic dust both on 9/11 and during the cleanup.[306]

We in the 9/11 community have a lot in common with the other victims of acts of terror and climate change, but the problem is, we're usually loath to admit it. There has always been a sense that we need to distinguish 9/11 from other tragedies so that we can establish ourselves as especially worthy of assistance. We didn't develop this mentality in a vacuum. We aren't just needlessly selfish. This was how politicians and strategists told us we'd have to be if we ever wanted to see a dime of funding come our way. The sense was, *Just because things should be different, it doesn't mean they always are.* Our political system provides almost no basic support, then leaves us all fighting for funding scraps. We had to own it.

The limited resources available made us competitive with each other too. Responders have, at various turns, quietly thrown the survivor community out the window when it's looked like funding wouldn't be forthcoming. Politicians have repeatedly done the same. And I get it.

Responders were sick and desperate for help, just like us. They needed what they needed. They had leverage we didn't have because America knew they existed. On the community side we have, in turn, played the 9/11 card to distinguish ourselves from other communities of victims. At a certain point when your community is sick and scared, you do what you have to do to get the funding you need.

It's not that there's a perfect system in some other country where competing interests don't jockey for attention and resources, but American disaster victims lose out in especially striking ways because we're often playing defense and asking for small funding bursts just to cover basic ongoing care. We don't get the luxury of focusing on specialized needs and specific resources, and when we do, it's to make our asks seem smaller and cheaper, not because they're the only help we need. This is a system that can only exist in a place where there is no baseline of basic, no cost, universal health care.

The problem is, there isn't much motivation to change any of this, at least inside the system. Treating disasters as distinct is convenient for a lot of people—people, for example, who are charged with figuring out how to actually sell new policy ideas or policy changes. During the 9/11 Health and Compensation Act's legislative process we were repeatedly told that nobody in Congress would agree to an entitlement program, because that sets a "dangerous" precedent. We were told to be very clear that there are limits to who qualifies for our programs that are scrupulously enforced. We were told to make sure our program could still shut the door on some people so the system wouldn't be upended.

The logic of this thinking is absurd. Events that lack the large-scale political resonance of 9/11 are still bad for the people dealing with them, even when they aren't politically expedient for the people using them. The social and economic havoc wreaked by the COVID-19 pandemic just on the heels of the Zadroga extension legislation has made that very clear. What we in the 9/11 community have in common with every other disaster victim (which, in this moment, might include everybody in America), regardless of whether their disaster was man-made or natural, big or small, accidental or intentional, is the need for an entitlement program. Health care *should* be something to which we are all already entitled. We shouldn't have had to sell our needs as special and unique, as if we aren't sure of that basic fact.

All this is to say that, at some point—and I don't know how to engineer that point—we all have to start focusing on the bigger prize. And that's not a special monitoring program for 9/11 survivors or responders. That prize is that every person in America gets access to meaningfully affordable or preferably free, baseline, high-quality, comprehensive health care so that having something treatable like asthma—whether it's caused by a disaster or just bad luck, whether it's being exasperated by an infectious pandemic or just run-of-the-mill air pollution—doesn't bankrupt or kill them. Every person in America should have care that's comprehensive enough that after an environmental disaster, victims can get cancer treatment *before* the specialized research identifying the unique risks they faced kicks in, comprehensive enough that they can find out that they are sick in the first place, long before somebody thinks to give them access to a screening appointment at a federal health program ten years later. As somebody who entered her twenties during a particularly disastrous time in America's health care system, I am well aware of the fact that all the fancy monitoring programs in the world don't help you if you don't yet have a diagnosis and can't afford to see a doctor to get one.

THE FACT THAT A large community at Ground Zero was so vulnerable to this treatment—to being overlooked after an event of massive political important like 9/11—should also lead us to think critically about why and how we, in apportioning public money in the piecemeal way that we do, value certain people's health and well-being over those of others.

Often in the 9/11 community, survivors—those of us who lived, worked, or went to school in Lower Manhattan—are overtly discussed as lesser victims, entitled to less care. Throughout the decades-long legislative process we were told this repeatedly, in no uncertain terms, often in a tone that read as, *Sorry to say it, but we all know it's the truth.* Don Lemon's booker knew it when she turned me away two hours before air so they could have a responder on instead. Our lead advocate knew it when he said, "She's speaking last, but she's speaking." My friend's wife, the one who told me I was insensitive for discussing 9/11's ongoing health aftermath because people had died on the day, she knew it too.

I probably sound bitter, but I don't really fault the people who said these things on our team. New Yorkers like straight talk, and our strategists wanted us to know the truth. We all knew how the story would play in the media. Survivors didn't do anything that contributed to the mythology around 9/11, so of course we couldn't be valuable. We didn't answer a call or run toward the danger. We weren't heroic. There is, in fact, very little to feel pride in as a survivor. We were lied to. We believed the lie, or, in my case at Stuyvesant, the adults in charge of us believed (or, depending on your point of view, exploited) the lie. Our health was put in danger. That's it. All we did was show up. Our story is, at best, neutral. At worst it's antagonistic to the warm and fuzzy feelings people want to bask in when thinking back on the great unity America experienced after 9/11.

On the other hand, the value conversation is important, because the value you're given as a victim in the American system determines who takes your complaint seriously, whether your needs are addressed with funding, whether you get press and outreach opportunities, and whether you get to hear your story validated by other voices. Why we survivors feel our inferiority so keenly is sort of a chicken-or-egg question—was it because we were repeatedly told, and shown, we were inferior or because we inherently understood the unspoken value system in America? Either way there's a larger conversation to have about why we, and everybody around us, seemed to inherently understand that we would be perceived this way. Why they offered us fewer benefits than responders in the final Zadroga package, requiring us to be sick before being screened, requiring our individual health coverage to cover the primary costs of care while responders' costs are covered in full by the program.[307] Why we knew we'd have to take that offer and be thankful we got it.

It should surprise nobody that the criteria we use to assess people's value as victims is reflective of the ways we assess value more broadly. Because of this, the criteria is often problematic. Cis, white, able-bodied men rule the roost in the best of times, and they rule the roost in the worst of times too. Perhaps this is why white communities get to be valuable victims more often than communities of color and rich communities get to be valuable victims more often than poor communities. Often those are one and the same. Sandy Hook's and Parkland's visibility after their tragic mass shootings may have resulted in a lot of media coverage, often framed as if the nation had just woken up to the scourge of gun violence, but African Americans between the ages of fifteen and twenty-nine are eighteen times more likely to die as a result of gun homicide than their white counterparts.[308] They are also two and a half times more likely to be murdered by the police, and though that statistic has been true for years, we've done very little to address the problem.[309] All of these layers play a role not just in who gets to be a victim at all but also who gets to speak for a diverse community when there's money on the line. As I've said, there's no reason to be surprised that it was a white, middle-class Stuyvesant grad who went to an expensive college who got put forth as the voice of a community that includes wealthy enclaves like Tribeca and Battery Park City but also Chinatown and other communities of color.

Still, in the case of 9/11, there's a bigger distinction between the responder and survivor coalitions, because the thing that really sets apart survivor advocates is that we are almost entirely female. Frankly, who else steps up when a whole community is in need? The responder advocates, by contrast, are mostly law enforcement and emergency services members and are mostly white and male. This, of course, isn't to say that there aren't great guys (and, periodically, people of color and women!) in that cohort. It's certainly not to suggest that many of them haven't been steadfast supporters of StuyHealth's work, of the survivor community, and that some didn't help echo my concerns to members of Congress and the press when they were loath to listen. It has, however, impacted a lot about the way our stories are received by political offices, the media, and the public. In 9/11 terms, to be a valuable victim, you had to be a "hero." Women don't have an easy time meeting that criteria.

The idea that heroes deserve health care, by the way, isn't inherently problematic. But if being a hero is what makes you deserving, then it matters that the way we define "hero" is gendered. It means that the way we define need is gendered. It means that the way we think about who *deserves* health care—because in America, health care is not a universal right—is gendered. 9/11's first responder population is almost 90 percent male.[310] The jobs that qualify people to meet the criteria for "heroic" are also vastly disproportionally male, as they are in jobs that are associated with physical power and size like police work and firefighting and construction. It still boggles my mind that on 9/11 there were only thirty women *in total* in the FDNY.[311] In fact, 9/11's EMT responders, which are a more diverse and vastly more female cohort,[312] got pushback when they wanted access to certain responder benefits despite their very clear lifesaving roles.[313]

This wide chasm in the public sentiment around the people who are affected and the people who are elevated as heroes is why the responder story had to be purposefully elevated to the exclusion of everybody else. When footage of Jon Stewart lambasting Congress at the 2019 VCF hearing went viral, Americans did not see any coverage of me a few seats down from him, nor any other women, even though our panel was half female. The fact that the four men and four women got seated by gender, with women up first and men as closers, was intentional—the order was a subject of much coded conversation and debate among the advocates and committee staff because they wanted to make sure the hearing made the news. The idea (and it was an effective one) was not articulated to me in so many words, but the implication was clear—let the men speak last because, no matter how impactful my or any other woman's story was going to be, female victims simply aren't seen as valuable enough to carry a story about heroes.

The complicated criteria we use to quantify victimhood extends far beyond the community's experience on and after 9/11, of course. We've all done a lot of #NeverForgetting since 9/11, and I know from experience that being the people who are routinely forgotten in the #NeverForget rhetoric takes a toll. What also takes a toll is that nobody uses #NeverForget rhetoric when it's only kids or women or people of color who are suffering. I've never heard anybody say #NeverForget Flint. Or #NeverForget that beyond Flint, thousands of rural communities in America lack access to clean water.[314] Or #NeverForget the fact that we lost twice as many women to domestic violence as we did soldiers to war during the incursions in Iraq and Afghanistan.[315] Or #NeverForget that Black COVID-19 victims are significantly more likely to die of the disease due to the underlying inequalities in our health care system.[316] Those situations are equally deserving of our memory and action.

As many responders have told me as we walked the halls of Congress, they were doing a job. They knew their job was dangerous. That's not to suggest that they should have been subjected to dangerous chemicals without their knowledge or asked to work without proper safety precautions or forced to lobby Congress for twenty years before securing permanent help. Of course not. It is, however, to suggest, that many of them saw that there was an inherently unequal element to how our stories were treated by the rest of America. They were rightfully glorified, but in the process, we were actively forgotten. The 9/11 survivor community often couldn't make as effective a case for itself because we couldn't meet criteria that were designed to exclude us.

I love the responders I fought beside for all these years, and I know that my classmates and I and the hundreds of thousands of other survivors downtown would have never gotten help without them, but at this point, twenty years down the line, I can't stand it when people say #NeverForget It never means "Let's never forget the full scope of the crisis." Half the time on Capitol Hill the people #NeverForgetting couldn't even remember the responders they spoke about so admiringly. We had to go into meetings with printouts of their tweets about 9/11 to remind them.

The forgetting is a vicious cycle too. The more a community is forgotten, the more its members absorb the message that they don't matter, the more they find themselves isolated, the more they have trouble getting data, the more they lack information about whether they're actually sick or affected, the more they fade from the collective national memory. The physical impacts of 9/11 happened in a small, relatively privileged part of a huge city, but the cycle of forgetting occurs in lots of other communities too. Communities with no political capital to spend—poor communities, communities of color, the kind of communities the American political system doesn't sympathize with—always get the short end of the stick after major crises. After Hurricane Maria hit in 2017, despite a death toll in the thousands, the US government claimed for months that only sixty-four people had died due to the storms.[317] They didn't bother to acquire or examine the real data, and if they didn't have the data, they didn't have a problem to solve. As a result, they dragged their feet getting emergency funding to the island in the middle of a major humanitarian crisis. Even more people died as a result.[318] It sounds familiar, because the same thing happened after Hurricane Katrina. Without data on the crisis, there is no visible problem to solve—but who is responsible for getting the data? In an ideal world, that's a role for government too. In the real world the responsibility usually falls on victims themselves.

If all of this isn't frustrating enough, there are also organizational disadvantages built into this system of victim value that can affect a community's ability to advocate for itself. At the starting level there are things as simple as finding advice about how to form a community group or nonprofit when you don't know where to begin. I winged it in that department for years because my issue wasn't high-profile enough.

Then, once you are at the level where Congress is considering legislation related to your issue, there is the question of whether that community group or nonprofit is allowed to fund lobbying activities and, if not, where to find a benefactor. I was delinquent there as well. For years I covered the costs of lobbying on 9/11 health issues independently because it was important and I could. That press conference in February 2019 was the first time that it occurred to me that I'd backed myself into a corner. I'd limited the time and resources I could spend organizing by not looking for donors. I was, fortunately, in a position where I could blow my budget to get to DC because I knew somebody would bail me out. That's the definition of privilege. Later, though, when that bailout was in the form of private money for travel, it had strings attached, and I had to make some hard choices that did not always feel like the best choices for the cause.

Once all of the criteria are met, communities also have to figure out how to overcome bureaucratic malaise. The systems that did ultimately get set up for us in the 9/11 community require constant monitoring, constant pushing, and therefore constantly engaged advocates who have to somehow find the time and resources to pay their rent while becoming experts in the intricacies of a deliberately complicated system.

I FELL INTO A severe depression in the fall of 2019, as soon as the VCF extension passed and the bulk of our political work was done. It lasted for a few months, and, despite what most people assumed, it was not prompted by the letdown in excitement or the fact that I no longer had Washington events to attend and had to settle into something like normal life. It was fine with me that I would have some time to spend at home.

The depression was caused by a different part of the natural shift that took place in that period, a shift in focus among the 9/11 health advocates. We had spent years, guns blazing on the political front, and then, suddenly, all we had left was to manage the services we had won. We'd been doing that all along while pursuing those other aims, but this time a general consensus emerged that we couldn't acknowledge what we hadn't won, specifically what services the survivor community hadn't gotten that the responder community had. That included our right to be monitored and our desire to see health studies address our needs so treatment for linked women's and developmental health conditions could be added to the list of covered services.[319] We were told they'd come eventually. Maybe. Either way, not worth the risk of raising a kerfuffle. Not worth the risk of complaining about a privilege we'd just acquired.

It started as an unspoken thing, but by September 2019 I was getting phone calls from other advocates warning me not to say specific things to the press. Things that, in some cases, I had already said publicly about where my cohort still lacked coverage. I'd mentioned to a reporter that people who were minors during the attack and cleanup deserved a proactive monitoring program, that we should not have to wait until we're already sick to get screened. I'd mentioned that developmental health concerns were not being adequately studied. I was, in response, repeatedly warned not to upset the apple cart—everything was now to be a small bureaucratic fight instead of a large political one. Our goals were no longer forward-thinking, they were maintenance. I had to understand that.

I didn't. For one thing, we were talking about maintenance at a time when we still had much to remedy. This was before the COVID-19 pandemic began, but health care protections for the general population were diminishing and care was becoming out of reach for many people like us. Even our own cohort's needs were shifting as we moved from our twenties to our thirties and began having kids and thinking about what that future entailed. Began thinking about the black cloud of health concerns hanging over our own futures. To be asked repeatedly not to voice any further concerns was very demoralizing after all the work we'd put in.

IN WRITING ABOUT THIS experience I've been reflecting a lot on why I got involved in this particular issue. After all, it required me to spend years steeped in an unpleasant memory, doing work that has sometimes felt like one frustration after another. What I've come to is that this was the only way to exercise agency in a situation in which I had none. In the moments that my agency has been being challenged, it has been unpleasant. In the moments in which that agency has worked to achieve something, it's been incredibly satisfying. In my darkest moments, it's been helpful to have something to push forward on. I'd recommend it. I can't say I'm self-aware enough to know why I had the energy to try it, but finding something to stand for in the middle of a huge, all-encompassing trauma is a good way to use the anxious energy an event like that generates.

Looking forward, I want my health care advocacy work to keep being satisfying, but to truly do what we need to do to protect me and people like me from further harm, we have to be willing to learn from past mistakes and we have to continue to make bigger asks. It took a decade of fighting for 9/11 survivors and responders to get a tiered health program that covers at least some of our needs. There is no similar program for the thousands of school shooting victims, the millions of people recovering from fires and floods, the absolute tragedy one hurricane can bring to a coastal community. There is no national health program to take care of all of us in the middle of a life-changing pandemic. We are, instead, waiting around for the victims of these disasters to ask for care even though we can extrapolate from the 9/11 experience, as well as disasters past, that they need it. That it would be valuable to all of us, when disaster visits us, to not have to ask for help in the first place. There's a reason the conversation around single-payer systems (or Medicare for All, as it's generally referred to in the US context) seems to pick up when we're at our most vulnerable.

Instead of waiting around or letting ourselves get drawn into a system that pits victims against each other, we should proactively attend to all of their unfortunately imminent problems—Flint's need for clean water, the need to pass some kind of gun control legislation, the need to wear masks to stop the further spread of COVID, as well as the problems that forthcoming disaster victims are sure to face down the road—and the never-ending health care costs that come with living through the aftermath of a crisis. Figuring out how to do this is, in part, the responsibility of victims like myself, who should take the victories we've won and lessons we've learned and start thinking broadly about how to help others like us. We should fight for their access to care as if it's our own community on the line, because in so many ways it actually is.

Most importantly, we should not allow political inertia to convince us that this isn't a practical or reasonable proposition. There are a lot of experts out there whose job it is to place what they feel are reasonable limits on people's agency for the sake of some larger agenda. What I've realized in the years since 2006, when I raised my head and decided, "I want to complain about this," is that you can't let other people dictate what's "reasonable." Asking for more might make their jobs harder, but that's not our problem. We can decide what's reasonable based on our experience and those forces, whether they be the political establishment or just the constant pull of inertia, can adjust.

As my mother always told me on our trips to Washington, we are stakeholders in our government. We own these systems. We can decide how they should work and whom they should work for. We should think broadly and act boldly because our systems can and should work for all of us.

HOW TO GET STARTED

can't say I consulted a lot of books or resources about how to be an activist when I was starting my work with StuyHealth. I made it up as I went along—I put my foot in my mouth fairly frequently (and probably still do). I knew nothing about fundraising or grants. I had never managed people or professional relationships. I had never even had a real job. Often, I would hear other people's opinions about how to best exercise my power as a voter, as an activist, as a community member, or just as an ornery person and assume they knew something that I didn't about my life, my skills, or my potential. Most of them didn't. A lot of them were underestimating me. Some didn't seem to recognize even the most basic things about where I could offer value and where I couldn't.

There are a lot of ways to become an activist. It's fine to volunteer with the big organizations, but you don't need the approval or involvement of a large national organization to do effective and meaningful work. A lot of effective community organizations start informally and inexpertly, led by people who have a burning need to do something and not much else to go on.

With that said, there are helpful things to know about how to approach advocacy and community work. It was a stroke of incredible luck that I had parents who were active in the community, as well as teachers who were invested in me and helped me develop my voice. I was brought to protests and meetings and events that taught me what advocacy can look like, where it can happen, and how to recognize its successes. I was one of the few American schoolkids who were offered a civics class in school, it was only as an elective, but it was valuable. Here are some things those mentors and role models and teachers taught me that helped me navigate my early organizing adventures.

Being an Active Citizen Begins with Some Basic Steps

You may have a cause you care about or a policy you want to change, but first you have to care about your vote. Register. Vote in every election, even if it's an off year and nothing splashy is on the ballot. Make sure your mom and BFF and cousins and even the people you hate vote.

Spend some time every day reading, watching, or listening to the news. Following the news will help you figure out which candidates and parties represent your views. Knowing what's going on will also stop you from being the person who says, "I know the American health care system sucks, but I don't know how to fix it." Most importantly, being up on the news will help you figure out which politicians are working on the issues you care about, what they're proposing, and what solutions you support.

Make informal activism a habit. Be the friend who keeps your circle informed and gets others to the polls, to protests, or to advocacy events. Help people look up their representatives so that when they have a problem you can give them the tools to solve it. I write voting guides for my friends for every election. If I run across anybody, from Lyft drivers to neighbors or family members, who can't figure out how to register to vote, get to the polls, or research their ballot, I help them work it out. I don't do that work on behalf of some big organization or under the banner of a "cause," I just do it because it seems like somebody should. It's still activism, and anybody can do it if they're familiar with the ways of Google.

Getting a Group Off the Ground

Find a specific cause. It's easy to feel overwhelmed by how many communities need help and how many systems need fixing. It's much less overwhelming, however, if you focus your energy on something specific. The more narrow and local the issue is, the easier it is to get traction and the attention of elected officials and community leaders. Smaller, community-based actions are what create and sustain bigger movements.

Find people to work with. Get friends involved in your issue. You may also find that activists or organizations are already working in your area of interest. If so, get in touch with them and find out where their work needs support. They may have ongoing or complementary work you can plug in to. If they don't, they may offer expertise or resources that bolster the work you're looking to do.

The most useful skill you can have as an activist or advocate is being a good storyteller. That also means being an effective writer. Once you have a cause, don't just post on social media and call it a day. Look for opportunities to submit op-eds and send letters to the newspaper. If a bill you're interested in is being heard, see if you can submit testimony. (There are a ton of resources online, varying by state and level of government, that will teach you how to do it.)

You can do a lot of this stuff for free. Fundraising is annoying, especially if you don't have friends or family with deep pockets. Often people will talk about it as if it's the first thing you need to consider. Funds are helpful, but, especially when working on local issues, there's a lot you can do without any sort of budget. It's free to have ideas, to post on social media. It's free to write letters and op-eds and to talk to the press. That's not to say that money isn't helpful. Travel is expensive. Events are expensive. Your time should be expensive (wouldn't that be nice?). Still, raising the profile of an issue isn't just about money. Don't let fundraising concerns hold you back. Work with the resources you have.

Dealing with Government

You can just walk into your representative's office. Don't take this to mean that you can organize a violent coup and invade the Capitol (I can't believe that needs to be said), but your legislators' offices are open to the public. At every level of government. In Washington, DC, in every state, and every city. It's by design, and it's so their constituents can visit them. It's wild how many people don't know that. Go visit your reps!

Introduce yourself to politicians if you see them around. People do this to them all day. If you have an issue you care about, you can tell them what you think about it on the street, in an elevator, or at a party. Be respectful, of course, but just because they are probably wearing suits doesn't mean they are your boss. They work for their district. If you're from their district, they work for you.

Learn the jargon. The book I routinely recommend when people ask for advocacy resources is not a how-to or an inspiring biography or a nonfiction story of David-versus-Goliath-level success, it's *The Beltway Bible* by Eliot

Nelson (Macmillan, 2016). It's a glossary of every ridiculous inside-baseball political term you'll ever hear on Capitol Hill and it's incredibly useful and, as a bonus, funny.

Talking to media is fun. But you should learn the basics of how to talk to the press. Know what it means to be "on" or "off" the record. Figure out which media reports on the kind of cause you're dealing with. Being a small-time activist often means being your own press agent.

Overall

Embrace the Occupy model. "Occupy" might be a dated reference, but it tends to surface when your life has revolved around an issue that was so long ago that there's already a museum devoted to it. I came of age in an era where being anti-war meant you'd be sent to volunteer for a large nonprofit that would ask you to sit alone and stuff envelopes for hours for no pay. Those experiences were so unpleasant, the "bosses" so condescending, the offices so dusty and depressing, that they stopped me from pursuing other social justice work later on. If you care about being involved in an issue but other activists are demanding that you contribute in ways that sound offensive, unappealing, or weirdly gendered (this happens a lot!), appoint yourself to be in charge of something else. The most important thing for the cause is that you make good use of the skills you bring to the table. If you're a great designer, design something. If you're social, appoint yourself in charge of recruiting. A lot of people drawn to politics crave authority, but don't let other people's power trips stop you from pursuing change on your terms.

Being an activist is an act of optimism. Sometimes people will claim that activists are just people who wanted to complain. Those are people without vision. Just trying to fix any of the zillions of issues people face that make their lives harder is inherently optimistic. Learn to spot the victories, even if they aren't perfect.

In general, plenty of well-meaning advice about how to advocate for a cause will fail you. Some of it won't be relevant to you. Pieces of it will be designed to exclude, not empower, you. Too much of it will be written in books that are hundreds of pages long and make it seem as though, without $1 million in seed money or Barack Obama's personal phone number or a doctorate in community organizing, you shouldn't bother pursuing political change in the first place. Or, perhaps, you'll read that you should direct your volunteer time and money toward somebody who does have those things and therefore knows better than you.

You can and should take all of that advice, along with everything I've written here, with a grain of salt. If there is an injustice you want to address, a community you want to help, a political figure you want to work for, you should just do what seems right to you. You know your experience, you know your community, and you know your skills. You are the expert. That's enough.

NOTES

1   Helen Kennedy, "Columbine High School Shootings Leave 15 Dead
    and 24 Injured in 1999," *New York Daily News,* April 15, 2015,
    https://www.nydailynews.com/news/national/high-school-bloodbathgun
    -toting-teens-kill-25-article-1.822951.

2   Josh Getlin, "Plan to Ban Jaywalking in N.Y. Gets Laugh," *Sun Sentinel,*
    January 17, 1998, https://www.sun-sentinel.com/news/fl-xpm-1998-01-17
    -9801160363-story.html.

3   Amanda Holpuch, "Columbine at 20: How School Shootings Became
    'Part of the American Psyche,'" *The Guardian*, April 17, 2019,
    https://www.theguardian.com/us-news/2019/apr/17/how-columbine
    -changed-america-20-year-anniversary-school-shootings.

4   Tom Hays, "AP Was There: The 1993 Bombing of the World Trade Center,"
    Associated Press, February 25, 2018, https://apnews.com/article/
    f4f1fd2b2d4b4a17b94ca7183fb65ba4.

5   Katrina Shakarian, "The History of New York City's Specialized High Schools,"
    Gotham Gazette, https://www.gothamgazette.com/government/5392-the
    -history-of-new-york-citys-special-high-schools-timeline; Robert D. McFadden
    with Eben Shapiro, "Finally, a Facade to Fit Stuyvesant: A High School of High
    Achievers Gets a High-Priced Home," *The New York Times*, September 8, 1992,
    https://www.nytimes.com/1992/09/08/nyregion/finally-facade-fit-stuyvesant-
    high-school-high-achievers-gets-high-priced-home.
    html?searchResultPosition=2.

6   Benjamin Mueller, William K. Rashbaum, and Al Baker, "Terror Attack Kills 8 and Injures 11 in Manhattan," *The New York Times*, October 31, 2017, https://www.nytimes.com/2017/10/31/nyregion/police-shooting-lower-manhattan.html.

7   "The Race for Mayor," *Gotham Gazette*, https://www.gothamgazette.com/searchlight2001/mayor1.html.

8   Ibid.

9   Abigail Deutsch, "Untitled," *The Spectator*, November 20, 2001, https://issuu.com/stuyspectator/docs/wtc.

10 Thankfully, I was able to confirm later that all of those students made it out safely.

11 Deutsch, *The Spectator*.

12 "Oklahoma City Bombing," History, FBI, accessed March 25, 2021, https://www.fbi.gov/history/famous-cases/oklahoma-city-bombing.

13 11septembervideos, "Bomb Threat Stuyvesant High School," YouTube video, 1:00, July 8, 2009, https://www.youtube.com/watch?v=ozMYlC-Tlb8.

14 "Ground Zero," History.com, August 13, 2010, https://www.history.com/topics/21st-century/ground-zero/.

15 "9/11: Cantor Fitzgerald Survival Story," BBC, September 11, 2011, https://www.bbc.com/news/av/uk-politics-14870543/9-11-cantor-fitzgerald-survival-story.

16 Jane Pae, "Painting for Peace," *The Spectator*, November 20, 2001, https://issuu.com/stuyspectator/docs/wtc.

17 Susan Ferraro, "EPA Chief Says Water, Air Are Safe," *New York Daily News*, September 14, 2001.

18 Anthony DePalma, "Ex-EPA Chief Defends Role in Response," *The New York Times*, June 26, 2007, https://www.nytimes.com/2007/06/26/nyregion/26whitman.html.

19 Jeremy P. Jacobs, "EPA Regulators Say They've Learned From 9/11 Blunders, But Critics Remain Unconvinced," *The New York Times*, September 9, 2011, https://archive.nytimes.com/www.nytimes.com/gwire/2011/09/09/09greenwire-epa-regulators-say-theyve-learned-from-911-blu-24494.html?pagewanted=all.

20 Stephen G. Bloom, "Lesson of a Lifetime," *Smithsonian Magazine*, September 2005, https://www.smithsonianmag.com/science-nature/lesson-of-a-lifetime-72754306/.

21 Ibid.

22 Ibid.

23 Susan Saulny and Andrew C. Revkin, "A Nation Challenged: Battery Park City; E.P.A. Says Air Is Safe, But Public Is Doubtful," *The New York Times*, October 6, 2001, https://www.nytimes.com/2001/10/06/nyregion/nation-challenged-battery-park-city-epa-says-air-safe-but-public-doubtful.html?searchResultPosition=7.

24 Elisabeth Bumiller, "A Nation Challenged: The Visit; Bush Tries to Reassure Children and Executives," *The New York Times*, October 4, 2001, https://www.nytimes.com/2001/10/04/nyregion/a-nation-challenged-the-visit-bush-tries-to-reassure-children-and-executives.html?searchResultPosition=12.

25 U.S. Congressman Jerrold Nadler, "White Paper: Lower Manhattan Air Quality," March 11, 2002, 3, https://nadler.house.gov/sites/nadler.house.gov/files/documents/epa%20white%20paper%20final%203_11.pdf.

26 Eric Lipton, "A Nation Challenged: The Scene; Returning to the Office on the First Monday Since the City Changed," *The New York Times*, September 18, 2001, https://www.nytimes.com/2001/09/18/nyregion/nation-challenged-scene-returning-office-first-monday-since-city-changed.html?searchResultPosition=2.

27 Ibid.

28 William N. Rom, "Environmental Policy and Public Health" (San Francisco: Wiley, 2011), 128.

29 Susan Saulny, "A Nation Challenged: Battery Park City; The Displaced Begin to Make Their Way Back Home," *The New York Times*, September 21, 2001, https://www.nytimes.com/2001/09/21/nyregion/nation-challenged-battery-park-city-displaced-begin-make-their-way-back-home.html?searchResultPosition=54.

30 Edward Wyatt, "A Nation Challenged: The Schools; Students Set to Return to Stuyvesant Near Ruins," *The New York Times*, October 9, 2001, https://www.nytimes.com/2001/10/09/nyregion/a-nation-challenged-the-schools-students-set-to-return-to-stuyvesant-near-ruins.html?searchResultPosition=32.

31 Kenneth R. Bazinet, "A Fight vs. Evil, Bush and Cabinet Tell U.S.," *New York Daily News,* September 17, 2001, https://web.archive.org/web/20100505200651/http://www.nydailynews.com/archives/news/2001/09/17/2001-09-17_a_fight_vs__evil__bush_and_c.html.

32 Lisa Marie Williams and Katie Worth, "A Tale of Two Schools," *The Village Voice*, December 18, 2001, https://www.villagevoice.com/2001/12/18/a-tale-of-two-schools/.

33 Carl Campanile, "Asbestos Fallout at Stuy High," *New York Post*, August 14, 2002, https://nypost.com/2002/08/14/asbestos-fallout-at-stuy-high/.

34 Irene Plagianos, "City to Revamp Stuyvesant High Auditorium Where 9/11 Dust Concerns Still Linger," DNAInfo, July 2, 2014, https://www.dnainfo.com/new-york/20140702/battery-park-city/city-revamp-stuyvesant-high-auditorium-where-911-dust-concerns-linger/.

35 Francesca Lyman, *Messages in The Dust: What Are the Lessons of the Environmental Health Response to the Terrorist Attacks of September 11?* (Denver: National Environmental Health Association, 2003), 31, https://www.iehaind.org/resources/pdf/messages_in_the_dust.pdf.

36 Abigail Deutsch, "Pressure from Parents, Change of Plans," *The Spectator*, October 2, 2001, https://issuu.com/stuyspectator/docs/wtc.

37 Ibid.

38 Ibid.

39 Carl Campanile, "School Sickens Me: Teach," *New York Post*, November 10, 2001, https://nypost.com/2001/11/10/school-sickens-me-teach/.

40 Laura Krug, "'A' for Air Quality," *The Spectator*, November 20, 2001, https://issuu.com/stuyspectator/docs/wtc.

41 Ibid.

42 Ibid.

43 Stuyvesant Parents' Association Environmental Health and Safety Committee, "Status Report," October 26, 2001.

44 Ibid.

45 Ibid.

46   Sarah Bartlett and John Patrarcha, *Schools of Ground Zero, Early Lessons Learned in Children's Environmental Health* (New York: American Public Health Association and Healthy Schools Network, 2002), 28.

47   Laura Krug, "'A' for Air Quality."

48   Susan Saulny and Andrew C. Revkin, "A Nation Challenged: Battery Park City; EPA Says Air Is Safe, But Public Is Doubtful."

49   Ibid.

50   Sarah Bartlett and John Patrarcha, *Schools of Ground Zero*, 14.

51   Yilu Zhao, "Students Get Back to Routine, But Sept. 11 Fears Linger," *The New York Times*, November 21, 2001, https://www.nytimes.com/2001/11/21/ nyregion/students-get-back-to-routine-but-sept-11-fears-linger. html?searchResultPosition=18.

52   Sarah Bartlett and John Patrarcha, 196–198.

53   E Baard, "The Dust May Never Settle," October 2, 2001, *The Village Voice*, accessed online at https://search.proquest.com/ docview/232286477?accountid=35804.

54   Kirk Johnson, "With Uncertainty Filling the Air, 9/11 Health Risks are Debated," *The New York Times*, February 8, 2002, https://www.nytimes.com/2002/02/08/ nyregion/with-uncertainty-filling-the-air-9-11-health-risks -are-debated.html?searchResultPosition=3.

55   David Klasfeld (Deputy Chancellor for Operations, Board of Education), "Letter to Students, Parents, and Staff of Stuyvesant," November 8, 2001.

56   Anne Raver, "Green Air Purifiers vs. Ground Zero," *The New York Times*, November 8, 2001, https://www.nytimes.com/2001/11/08/garden/human -nature-green-air-purifiers-vs-ground-zero.html.

57   "Mysterious Bonus Makes Rich NYC Schools Richer, Critics Say," WNYC News, November 8, 2017, https://www.wnyc.org/story/ mysterious-bonus-makes-rich-nyc-schools-richer-critics-say/.

58   Wayne Barrett with special research assistance by Alexandra Kahan, "Rudy Giuliani's Five Big Lies About 9/11," *The Village Voice*, July 31, 2007, https:// www.villagevoice.com/2007/07/31/rudy-giulianis-five-big-lies-about-911/.

59   Ibid.

60   Ibid.

324 SOME KIDS LEFT BEHIND

61 Ibid.

62 John M. Glionna, "At Giuliani Pad, Towels Say 'His', 'His,' and 'His.'" *LA Times*, September 2, 2001, https://www.latimes.com/archives/la-xpm-2001-sep-02 -mn-41294-story.html

63 U.S. Congress, *Public Law 107– 40*, 107th Congress, September 18, 2001, https://www.congress.gov/107/plaws/publ40/PLAW-107publ40.pdf.

64 "The US War in Afghanistan, 1999–2020," Council on Foreign Relations, accessed March 25, 2021, https://www.cfr.org/timeline/us-war-afghanistan.

65 "'You are either with us or against us,'" CNN, November 6, 2001, https://edition.cnn.com/2001/US/11/06/gen.attack.on.terror/.

66 Stephen D. Reese and Seth C. Lewis, "Framing the War on Terror: The Internalization of Policy in the US Press," *Journalism 10*, no.6 (2009): 777–779.

67 David E. Sanger, "The State of the Union: The Overview, Bush, Focusing on Terrorism, Says Secure U.S. Is Top Priority," *The New York Times*, January 30, 2002, https://www.nytimes.com/2002/01/30/us/state-union-overview-bush -focusing-terrorism-says-secure-us-top-priority.html.

68 Andrew Glass, "President Bush Cites 'Axis of Evil,' January 29, 2002," Politico, January 29, 2019, https://www.politico.com/story/2019/01/29/ bush-axis-of-evil-2002-1127725.

69 Ibid.

70 Jonathan Stein and Tim Dickinson, "Lie by Lie: A Timeline of How We Got into Iraq," *Mother Jones*, September 2006, https://motherjones.com/ politics/2011/12/leadup-iraq-war-timeline/.

71 "Hate Crime Reports Up in Wake of Terrorist Attack," CNN, September 17, 2001, https://web.archive.org/web/20100620204632/ http://archives.cnn.com/2001/US/09/16/gen.hate.crimes/.

72 Stuyvesant Parents' Association Environmental Health and Safety Committee, "Report to Parents," February 4, 2002.

73 Ibid.

74 Ibid.

75 Ibid.

76 Ibid.

77 Ibid.

78 Sarah Bartlett and John Patrarcha, *Schools of Ground Zero, Early Lessons Learned in Children's Environmental Health*, 29.

79 Stuyvesant Parents' Association Environmental Health and Safety Committee, "Report to Parents."

80 David Klasfeld (Deputy Chancellor for New York City Board of Education), "Letter to the Parents and Staff of Stuyvesant High School," February 7, 2002.

81 Ibid.

82 Stuyvesant Parents' Association Environmental Health and Safety Committee, "Response to February 7 Letter from Deputy Chancellor Klasfeld," undated.

83 "Statement from Executive Board Members Opposed to Legal Action Against the BOE," undated.

84 U.S. Congress, Senate, Committee on Environment and Public Works, *Air Quality in New York City after the September 11, 2001 Attacks*, 107th Congress, 2nd sess., 2002, 132, https://www.google.com/books/edition/Air_Quality_in_New_York_City_After_the_S/-c1MAQAAMAAJ?hl=en&gbpv=0.

85 Philip J. Landrigan, M.D., M. Sc., Mount Sinai School of Medicine, "Letter to Stuyvesant High School Parents, Staff, and Community," February 20, 2002.

86 Ibid.

87 Sarah Bartlett and John Patrarcha, *Schools of Ground Zero*, 218.

88 Sarah Bartlett and John Patrarcha, 30.

89 Bartlett and Patrarcha, appendix.

90 "Ceremony Closes 'Ground Zero' Cleanup," CNN, May 30, 2002, http://edition.cnn.com/2002/US/05/30/rec.wtc.cleanup/.

91 David W. Dunlap, "10 Years after 9/11 Deutsche Bank Tower Vanishes," January 12, 2011, https://cityroom.blogs.nytimes.com/2011/01/12/ten-years-after-911-the-wounded-deutsche-bank-tower-vanishes/.

92 Michael R. Gordon, "After the War: Preliminaries; US Air Raids in '02 Prepared for War in Iraq," *The New York Times*, July 20, 2003, https://www.nytimes.com/2003/07/20/world/after-the-war-preliminaries-us-air-raids-in-02-prepared-for-war-in-iraq.html.

93 "Full Text: In Cheney's Words," *The New York Times*, August 26, 2002, https://www.nytimes.com/2002/08/26/international/middleeast/full-text-in-cheneys-words.html.

94 "Bush's UN Speech: Full Text," BBC, September 13, 2002, http://news.bbc.co.uk/2/hi/middle_east/2254712.stm.

95 "Press Release for the Join Resolution for the Use of Force Authorization Against Iraq," White House Archive, October 2, 2002, https://web.archive.org/web/20021102072524/http://www.whitehouse.gov/news/releases/2002/10/20021002-2.html.

96 "Chronology: The Evolution of the Bush Doctrine," *Frontline*, PBS, accessed April 5, 2021, https://www.pbs.org/wgbh/pages/frontline/shows/iraq/etc/cron.html.

97 James Love, "Who Voted to Authorize Force in Iraq October 2002?" Huffington Post, February 8, 2008, https://www.huffpost.com/entry/who-voted-to-authorize-fo_b_85652?guccounter=1&guce_referrer=aHR0cHM6Ly93d3cuZ29vZ2xlLmNvbS8&guce_referrer_sig=AQAAAMrQF0_AxTV7VDEpCyxMR9QZd3Ykap7HzglccCPGxNTfNF67E-gehg3_SxM-o4tEowrKirRRGmPk4Anegu8Yq2emhmQHiUfFEPfUlZJknovKT98sVe6QJSLiJDY1adl_VQdsnEsD-l2xMWifInxM0fXT5tbbKrFX-_9CkJ7QzTM0.

98 "Cities jammed in worldwide protest of war in Iraq," CNN, February 16, 2003, http://www.cnn.com/2003/US/02/15/sprj.irq.protests.main/.

99 "Cities jammed in worldwide protest of war in Iraq," CNN.

100 Paul Blumenthal, "The Largest Protest Ever Was 15 Years Ago. The Iraq War Isn't Over. What Happened?" Huffington Post, February 15, 2018, https://www.huffpost.com/entry/what-happened-to-the-antiwar-movement_n_5a860940e4b00bc49f424ecb.

101 "Bush Declares War," CNN, March 19, 2002, https://www.cnn,com/2003/US/03/19/sprj.irq.int.bush.transcript/.

102 Leslie Eaton, "Thousands March in Manhattan Against War," *The New York Times*, March 22, 2003, https://www.nytimes.com/2003/03/22/international/worldspecial/thousands-march-in-manhattan-against-war.html.

103 "EPA's Response to the World Trade Center Collapse: Challenges, Successes, and Areas for Improvement," Report No. 2003-P-00012, August 21, 2003, https://www.epa.gov/sites/production/files/2015-12/documents/wtc_report_20030821.pdf,

104 *We Count: Documenting the 9/11 Health Crisis Eight Years Later* (New York: 9/11 Environmental Action and Beyond Ground Zero, 2009), 1, https:// takerootjustice.org/wp-content/uploads/2019/06/wecount_sept09.pdf.

105 The New York City Department of Health and Mental Hygiene, "City Health Information," *CME Activity Inside and Online* 4, vol. 28 (July 2009): 29–40, https://www1.nyc.gov/assets/doh/downloads/pdf/chi/chi28-4.pdf.

106 Pauline A. Thomas et al., "Respiratory and Other Health Effects Reported in Children Exposed to the World Trade Center Disaster of 11 September 2001," *Environmental Health Perspectives* 10, 116 (October 2008): https://www.ncbi.nlm.nih.gov/pmc/articles/PMC2569099/.

107 "WTC Health Registry," NYC 9/11 Health Website, https://www1.nyc.gov/ site/911health/index.page.

108 "World Trade Center Registry Questionnaire," 5, https://www1.nyc.gov/ assets/911health/downloads/pdf/wtc/wtc-questionnaire.pdf.

109 "Who Is Enrolled," NYC 9/11 Health Website, https://www1.nyc.gov/ site/911health/about/who-is-enrolled.page.

110 Ibid.

111 Jim Dwyer, "In Day of Mass Arrests, Divergent Version of Events," *The New York Times*, August 29, 2007, https://www.nytimes.com/2007/08/29/ nyregion/29about.html.

112 "New York to Pay $17.9 Million to 2004 Republican Convention Protesters," CNN, January 15, 2014 https://www.cnn.com/2014/01/15/politics/ new-york-republican-convention-settlement/index.html.

113 Jen Chung, "15 Years Ago, Protesters Took Over NYC During the Republican National Convention," Gothamist, August 30, 2019, https://gothamist.com/ news/15-years-ago-protesters-took-over-nyc-during-2004-republican-national -convention.

114 Jim Dwyer, "City Police Spied Broadly Before G.O.P. Convention," *The New York Times*, March 25, 2007, https://www.nytimes.com/2007/03/25/ nyregion/25infiltrate.html?pagewanted=all.

115 "New York to Pay $17.9 Million to 2004 Republican Convention Protesters," CNN.

116 Maggie Fox, "What Are Pre-Existing Conditions, and What Would the GOP Bill Do?" NBC, May 4, 2017, https://www.nbcnews.com/health/health-care/what-are-pre-existing-conditions-what-would-gop-bill-do-n754836.

117 Jennifer Pahre, "A Brief History of Health Care and Coverage for Pre-Existing Conditions," Illinois Public Media, August 7, 2017, https://will.illinois.edu/legalissuesinthenews/program/a-brief-history-of-health-care-and-coverage-for-pre-existing-medical-condit.

118 U.S. Congress, House, "Memorandum: Coverage Denials for Pre-Existing Conditions in the Individual Health Insurance Market," Committee on Energy and Commerce, 111th Cong., October 12, 2010, https://oversight.house.gov/sites/democrats.oversight.house.gov/files/documents/Memo-Coverage-Denials-Individual-Market-2010-10-12.pdf.

119 Ibid.

120 "Rape and Domestic Violence Could be Pre-existing Conditions," CNN, May 4, 2017, https://www.cnn.com/2017/05/04/health/pre-existing-condition-rape-domestic-violence-insurance/index.html.

121 Bill Hutchinson, "'Your Baby Is Too Fat': Insurer Denies Baby Alex Lange Coverage Because of Weight," *New York Daily News*, October 12, 2009, https://www.nydailynews.com/life-style/health/baby-fat-insurer-denies-baby-alex-lange-coverage-weight-article-1.381092.

122 U.S. Office of the Legislative Council, House, *Compilation of Patient Protection and Affordable Care Act*, HR3590, 111th Cong., 2nd sess., May 1, 2010, 13–137, 198–264, 471–503.

123 Peter Newell and Allan Baumgarten, *The Big Picture: Private and Public Health Insurance Markets in New York* (New York: United Hospital Fund, 2009), 104, https://info.nystateofhealth.ny.gov/sites/default/files/insurance_markets_in_ny.pdf.

124 Newell and Baumgarten, 5.

125 Deborah Reidy Kelch, *Insurance Markets: Rules Governing California's Individual Insurance Market* (Oakland: California Health Care Foundation). Revised April 2005, 4, https://www.chcf.org/wp-content/uploads/2017/12/PDF-RulesGoverningCAIndividualInsuranceMarket.pdf.

126 Stephen Smith, "Tale of the Walking Dead," CBS, February 23, 2006, https://www.cbsnews.com/news/tale-of-the-walking-dead/.

127 Julia Preston, "Public Misled on Air Quality After 9/11 Attack, Judge Says," *The New York Times*, February 3, 2006, https://www.nytimes.com/2006/02/03/nyregion/public-misled-on-air-quality-after-911-attack-judge-says.html.

128 Kareen Fahim, "Detective's Death Tied to Ground Zero Fumes," *The New York Times*, April 12, 2006, https://www.nytimes.com/2006/04/12/nyregion/detectives-death-tied-to-ground-zero-fumes.html.

129 Rossana Shokrian, "9/11 Workers Get Expanded Benefits in N.Y.," CNN, August 15, 2006, https://www.cnn.com/2006/US/08/15/911.health.benefits/index.html.

130 Mike Kelly, "'Mea Culpa Mike' Bloomberg's History of Apologizing for Gaffes Has NJ Connection," NorthJersey.com, February 21, 2020, https://www.northjersey.com/story/news/columnists/mike-kelly/2020/02/21/michael-bloomberg-has-habit-taking-back-dumb-statements/4823484002/.

131 Stephen Smith, "ME Claims 9/11 Cop Died from Drug Misuse," CBS, October 24, 2007, https://www.cbsnews.com/news/me-claims-9-11-cop-died-from-drug-misuse/.

132 Melissa Grace, "City Says Drug Use, Not Dust, Killed 9/11 Hero James Zadroga," *New York Daily News*, October 26, 2007, https://www.nydailynews.com/news/city-drug-not-dust-killed-9-11-hero-james-zadroga-article-1.232695.

133 Ibid.

134 Carla Nordstrom, "Why We Voted No," *The New York Times*, December 16, 1995, https://www.nytimes.com/1995/12/16/opinion/why-we-voted-no.html.

135 Nicholas Carlson, "At Last—The Full Story of How Facebook Was Founded," Business Insider, March 5, 2010, https://www.businessinsider.com/how-facebook-was-founded-2010-3.

136 Lila Nordstrom, "Open Letter," StuyHealth, March 31, 2006, http://stuyhealth.blogspot.com/2006/03/open-letter.html.

137 Ibid.

138 "Richard Ben-Veniste," Mayer Brown, accessed March 25, 2021, https://www.mayerbrown.com/en/people/b/benveniste-richard?tab=overview.

139 Sarah Bartlett and John Patrarcha, *Schools of Ground Zero*, 30.

140 National Commission on Terrorist Attacks upon the United States, "9/11 Commission Convenes, Names Executive Director," Archive, January 27, 2003, https://govinfo.library.unt.edu/911/press/pr_2003-01-27.htm.

141 Clemmy Manzo, "Grandmas Unite Against Injustice: Raging Grannies," Atlas of the Future, January 27, 2020, https://atlasofthefuture.org/project/raging-grannies/.

142 Carole Roy, "The Irreverent Raging Grannies: Humour As Protest," *Canadian Woman Studies* 25, no. 3,4 (2006): 141–148, https://cws.journals.yorku.ca/index.php/cws/article/viewFile/5901/5090.

143 "About Norman Siegel," The Law Offices of Siegel Teitelbaum & Evans, LLP, accessed March 25, 2021, http://stellp.com/nsiegel.html.

144 Kristen Lombardi, "Some Kids Left Behind," *The Village Voice*, September 5, 2006, https://www.villagevoice.com/2006/09/05/some-kids-left-behind/.

145 Office of the Mayor, "Mayor Bloomberg Announces Comprehensive Citywide Effort to Address 9/11 World Trade Center Health-related Issues," September 5, 2006, https://webcache.googleusercontent.com/search?q=cache:-Qzy8SaSoUcJ:https://www1.nyc.gov/office-of-the-mayor/news/319-06/mayor-bloomberg-comprehensive-citywide-effort-address-9-11-world-trade-center+&cd=1&hl=en&ct=clnk&gl=us&client=safari#/2.

146 Carl Campanile, "Workers Battle for 9/11 Suit," *New York Post*, June 22, 2006, https://nypost.com/2006/06/22/workers-battle-for-911-suit/.

147 Ibid.

148 "Recovery Snapshot: LMDC Residential Grant Program," US Department of Housing and Urban Development, https://www.hud.gov/sites/documents/DOC_22580.PDF.

149 Ibid.

150 Ibid.

151 "History," World Trade Center Health Program, Centers for Disease Control and Prevention, December 30, 2019, https://www.cdc.gov/wtc/history.html.

152 Anna Nowogrodzki, "Inequality in Medicine," *Nature* 550, S18–S19, 2017, https://doi.org/10.1038/550S18a.

153 Ibid.

154 Nowogrodzki.

155 Caroline Chen and Riley Wong, "Black Patients Miss Out on Promising Cancer Drugs," ProPublica, September 18, 2019, https://www.propublica.org/article/black-patients-miss-out-on-promising-cancer-drugs.

156 Michael W. Sodjing, M.D. et al., "Racial Bias in Pulse Oximetry Measurement," Letter to the Editor, *New England Journal of Medicine*, December 17, 2020, https://www.nejm.org/doi/full/10.1056/NEJMc2029240.

157 Stephen Stock, Robert Campos, and Michael Horn, "Experts Track Data to Reduce Police Violence," NBC Bay Area, June 4, 2020, *https://www.nbcbayarea. com/investigations/experts-track-data-to-reduce-police-violence/2303032/*.

158 Kristen Lombardi, "Some Kids Left Behind," *The Village Voice*.

159 Anthony DePalma, "Bloomberg Urges More Aid for Those Ailing After 9/11," *The New York Times*, February 14, 2007, https://www.nytimes. com/2007/02/14/nyregion/14health.html.

160 U.S. Congress, House, *9/11 Comprehensive Health Benefits Act of 2006*, HR 6046, 109th Congress, 1st sess., introduced September 7, 2006, https://www.congress.gov/bill/109th-congress/house-bill/6046/summary/.

161 Ibid.

162 Angela Fischer, email forwarded to Lila Nordstrom, January 27, 2007.

163 Carrie Melago, "Hil Joins Students' Fight for Stuy High 9/11 Tests," *New York Daily News*, October 13, 2006, https://www.nydailynews.com/archives/news/ hil-joins-students-fight-9-11-tests-article-1.646055.

164 Office of Rep. Carolyn B. Maloney, "9/11 Responders to Attend State of the Union Address with Gallery Passes Provided by N.Y. Senators, Reps.," January 22, 2007, https://maloney.house.gov/media-center/ press-releases/911-responders-attend-state-union-address-gallery-passes- provided-ny-senators-reps.

165 Edward Mills, email to author, "Monday, 1/22: Ground Zero News Conference with Ailing 9/11 Responders Attending State of the Union Address," January 18, 2007.

166 "Hillary Clinton Launches White House Bid: 'I'm In,'" CNN, January 22, 2007, https://www.cnn.com/2007/POLITICS/01/20/clinton.announcement/ index.html.

167 "Close Up Washington DC," accessed March 25, 2021, https://www.closeup.org/.

168 Dan Barry and Sheera Frenkel, "'Be There! Will Be Wild!': Trump All But Circled the Date," *The New York Times*, January 6, 2021, https://www.nytimes.com/ 2021/01/06/us/politics/capitol-mob-trump-supporters.html.

169 Francis X. Clines and Steven Lee Myers, "Attack on Iraq: The Overview; Impeachment Vote in House Delayed as Clinton Launches Iraq Air Strike, Citing Military Need to Move Swiftly," *The New York Times*, December 17, 1998, https://www.nytimes.com/1998/12/17/world/attack-iraq-overview -impeachment-vote-house-delayed-clinton-launches-iraq-air.html.

170 "About the September 11th Victim Compensation Fund," The United States Department of Justice, accessed March 25, 2021, https://www.justice.gov/ civil/vcf.

171 Catherine Kim, "The Battle over Expanding the September 11th Victim Compensation Fund, Explained," Vox, July 29, 2019, https://www.vox. com/2019/6/20/18691670/ jon-stewart-9-11-september-11th-victim-compensation-fund-explained.

172 Gabriela Schulte, "Poll: 60 Percent of Voters Support Medicare for All," The Hill, April 24, 2020, https://thehill.com/hilltv/what-americas-thinking/494602- poll-69-percent-of-voters-support-medicare -for-all.

173 Edward Mills, PDF attachment in email to author, March 13, 2007.

174 U.S. Congress, House of Representatives, Subcommittee on Government Management, Organization, and Procurement, Committee on Oversight and Government Reform, *Continuation of 9/11 Health Effects: Environmental Impacts for Residents and Responders*, 110th Congress, 1st sess., April 23, 2007, 15, https://www.govinfo.gov/content/pkg/CHRG-110hhrg40872/pdf/ CHRG-110hhrg40872.pdf.

175 Andy Broll, "How Occupy Wall Street Really Got Started," *Mother Jones*, October 17, 2011, https://www.motherjones.com/politics/2011/10/ occupy-wall-street-international-origins/.

176 Ben Davis, "How a Canadian Culture Magazine Helped Spark Occupy Wall Street," Blouin Artinfo, September 21, 2012.

177 Andy Broll, "How Occupy Wall Street Really Got Started."

178 Anthony DePalma, "Representatives Join Forces to Push New 9/11 Medical Bill," *The New York Times*, September 8, 2007, https://www.nytimes.com/ 2007/09/08/nyregion/08compensate.html.

179 Centers for Disease Control and Prevention, "CDC Awards $10 Million to New York Health and Hospitals Corporation to Provide Health Services to Residents, Other Community Members Affected by 9/11 Attack," News Release

(September 30, 2008), https://www.cdc.gov/media/pressrel/2008/r080930.htm.

180 Lila Nordstrom, "The Dust That Hasn't Settled," *The Guardian*, September 11, 2008, https://www.theguardian.com/commentisfree/cifamerica/2008/sep/11/uselections2008.september11.

181 Lila Nordstrom, "Lessons from 9/11 for the Gulf Oil Spill," *The Guardian*, June 17, 2010, https://www.theguardian.com/commentisfree/cifamerica/2010/jun/17/bp-oil-spill-september11.

182 U.S. Congress, House, James Zadroga 9/11 Health and Compensation Act of 2010, HR 847, 11th Congress, 2nd sess., introduced in House February 4, 2009, https://www.congress.gov/bill/111th-congress/house-bill/847; Congressional Budget Office, "Letter to Committee of Budget of US House," July 28, 2010, https://www.cbo.gov/sites/default/files/111thcongress-2009-2010/costestimate/hr84700.pdf.

183 Claudia Cruz, "9/11 Health Bill Loses Long Term Support," QNS, February 9, 2010, https://qns.com/2010/02/911-health-bill-loses-long-term-support/.

184 Ibid.

185 Meredith Kolodner, "Bloomberg Hails President Obama's Support of Zadroga Health Bill," *New York Daily News*, August 20, 2010, https://www.nydailynews.com/new-york/bloomberg-hails-president-obama-support-zadroga-9-11-health-bill-article-1.204970.

186 William Kormos, M.D., "When Does Long-term Acid Reflux Become a Serious Issue?" *Harvard Men's Health Watch* (Cambridge: Harvard Health Publishing, 2017), "https://www.health.harvard.edu/digestive-health/when-does-long-term-acid-reflux-become-a-serious-issue.

187 Raymond Hernandez, "Senate Passes 9/11 Health Bill as Republicans Back Down," *The New York Times*, December 22, 2010, https://www.nytimes.com/2010/12/23/nyregion/23health.html.

188 Among friends I am notorious for my love of great filibuster stories. My favorite remains Sen. Huey Long's classic 1935 filibuster, a fifteen-hour petty joyride through laughter, tears, Shakespeare, and recipes for fried oysters and other southern classics. Long began the filibuster not to protect the American people from some great foe but to prevent some of his political enemies from getting cushy government jobs at the National Recovery Administration. He was assassinated only a few months later, so he never got to break his own record, but

his thoughts on oysters remain one of his most important legacies. Michael Wertheim, "Here's a Senator's Recipe for Southern Fried Oysters, as Read During a 15-Hour Filibuster in 1935," Vice, October 11, 2011, https://www.vice.com/en_us/article/ezzzm7/heres-a-senators-recipe-for-southern-fried-oysters-as-read-during-a-15-hour-filibuster-in-1935.

189 Michael Cooper, "G.O.P. Senate Victory Stuns Democrats," *The New York Times*, January 19, 2010, https://www.nytimes.com/2010/01/20/us/politics/20election.html.

190 Ezra Klein, "Whatever Happened to the Public Option?" *The Washington Post*, March 23, 2013, https://www.washingtonpost.com/news/wonk/wp/2013/03/22/whatever-happened-to-the-public-option/.

191 John Baldoni, "John Feal Teaches Us What It Means to Serve Others," *Forbes*, September 12, 2017, https://www.forbes.com/sites/johnbaldoni/2017/09/12/john-feal-teaches-us-what-it-means-to-serve-others/?sh=57a567067e33.

192 Kate Phillips, "Senate Confirms Clinton as Secretary of State," *The New York Times*, January 21, 2009, https://thecaucus.blogs.nytimes.com/2009/01/21/senate-debates-clinton-confirmation/.

193 Javier C. Hernandez, Danny Hakim, and Nicholas Confessore, "Paterson Announces Choice of Gillibrand for Senate Seat," *The New York Times*, January 23, 2009, https://www.nytimes.com/2009/01/24/nyregion/24choice.html?ref=nyregion.

194 Raymond Hernandez, "Republicans Block U.S. Health Aid for 9/11 Workers," *The New York Times*, December 9, 2010, https://www.nytimes.com/2010/12/10/nyregion/10health.html.

195 Bill Carter and Brian Stelter, "In 'Daily Show' Role on 9/11 Bill, Echoes of Murrow," *The New York Times*, December 26, 2010, https://www.nytimes.com/2010/12/27/business/media/27stewart.html.

196 Ibid.

197 Ibid.

198 Robert D. McFadden, "Tom Coburn, the 'Dr. No' of Congress, Dead at 72," *The New York Times*, March 28, 2020, https://www.nytimes.com/2020/03/28/us/tom-coburn-dead.html

199 Cameron Joseph, "How Gillibrand Defied the Odds to Get First Responders Long-Awaited Help," Talking Points Memo, February 4, 2019, https://talkingpointsmemo.com/dc/kirsten-gillibrand-james-zadroga-september-11

200 Robert D. McFadden, "Tom Coburn, the 'Dr. No' of Congress, Dead at 72."

201 U.S. Congress, *An Act to Amend the Public Health Service Act to Extend and Improve Protections and Services to Individuals Directly Impacted by the Terrorist Attack in New York City on September 11, 2001, and for Other Purposes*, Public Law 111-347, Sec. 3321, 111th Cong., January 2, 2011, https://www.congress.gov/111/plaws/publ347/PLAW-111publ347.pdf.

202 Caroline Bankoff, "What We Know About How 9/11 Has Affected New Yorkers' Health, 15 Years Later," *New York* magazine, September 10, 2016, https://nymag.com/intelligencer/2016/09/15-years-later-how-has-9-11-affected-new-yorkers-health.html.

203 Joe Murphy et al., "Measuring and Maximizing Coverage in the World Trade Center Health Registry," *Statistics in Medicine* (Hoboken: John Wiley & Sons, 2007), http://www.nyc.gov/html/doh/wtc/downloads/pdf/wtc/wtc-article-20070207.pdf.

204 Cameron Joseph, "How Gillibrand Defied the Odds to Get *9/11 First Responders Long-Awaited Help*," Talking Points Memo, February 4, 2019, https://talkingpointsmemo.com/dc/kirsten-gillibrand-james-zadroga-september-11

205 Steve Koronaki, "What 'Don't Ask, Don't Tell' Did for Kirsten Gillibrand," Politico, December 20, 2010, https://www.politico.com/states/new-york/city-hall/story/2010/12/what-dont-ask-dont-tell-did-for-kirsten-gillibrand-067223.

206 Shane Goldmacher and Matt Flegenheimer, "Kirsten Gillibrand, Long a Champion of Women, Finds the Nation Joining Her," *The New York Times*, December 16, 2017, https://www.nytimes.com/2017/12/16/us/politics/senator-kirsten-gillibrand-trump-women-sexual-harassment.html.

207 Ibid.

208 Jesse Lee, "Photo: President Obama Signs the James Zadroga 9/11 Health and Compensation Act," Obama White House Archives (blog), January 2, 2011, https://obamawhitehouse.archives.gov/blog/2011/01/02/photo-president-obama-signs-james-zadroga-911-health-and-compensation-act.

209 Jen Chung, "Stuyvesant Alums Thwarted in Effort to Remembered 9/11 at High School," Gothamist, September 2, 2011, https://gothamist.com/news/stuyvesant-alums-thwarted-in-effort-to-remember-911-at-high-school.

210 Ibid.

211 Department of Health and Human Services, "Patient Protection and Affordable Care Act: Preexisting Condition Exclusions, Lifetime and Annual Limits, Rescissions, and Patient Protections," *Federal Register* 75, no. 123 (June 28, 2010): 37188, https://www.govinfo.gov/content/pkg/FR-2010-06-28/pdf/2010-15278.pdf.

212 "Average Individual Health Insurance Premiums Increased 99% Since 2013, the Year Before Obamacare, & Family Premiums Increased 140%, According to eHealth.com Shopping Data," eHealth, January 23, 2017, https://news.ehealthinsurance.com/news/average-individual-health-insurance-premiums-increased-99-since-2013-the-year-before-obamacare-family-premiums-increased-140-according-to-ehealth-com-shopping-data.

213 Dan Mangan, "Obamacare's Crushing Cost to Some Families: 49 Percent Price Hike Since 2014, Premiums of $14,300," CNBC, May 11, 2017, https://www.cnbc.com/2017/05/11/these-folks-dont-get-obamacare-subsidies-now-and-it-is-really-costing-them.html.

214 "Frequently Asked Questions," World Trade Center Health Program, February 11, 2021, https://www.cdc.gov/wtc/faq.html.

215 Graison Dangor, "'Mental Health Parity' Is Still an Elusive Goal in U.S. Insurance Coverage," NPR, June 7, 2019, https://www.npr.org/sections/health-shots/2019/06/07/730404539/mental-health-parity-is-still-an-elusive-goal-in-u-s-insurance-coverage.

216 Caroline Bankoff, "What We Know About How 9/11 Has Affected New Yorkers' Health, 15 Years Later."

217 Gary S. Becker, "The Painful Political Truth about Medical Research," Bloomberg, July 29, 1996, https://www.bloomberg.com/news/articles/1996-07-28/the-painful-political-truth-about-medical-research.

218 U.S. Congress, House, *James Zadroga 9/11 Health and Compensation Reauthorization Act*, H.R. 1786, 114th Cong., 2nd sess., introduced in House April 14, 2015, https://www.govtrack.us/congress/bills/114/hr1786.

219 Jonathan Lemire, "Jon Stewart, Firefighters Rally in D.C. for 9/11 Responder Benefits," NBC New York, September 16, 2015, https://www.nbcnewyork.com/

news/local/jon-stewart-politicians-firefighters-rally-on-capital-hill
-reauthorize-zadroga-bill-911/672313/.

220 Citizens for the Extension of the James Zadroga Act, "Mr. Stewart Goes to
     Washington....Citizens for the Extension of the James Zadroga Act & 9/11
     Responder/Advocate John Feal Announce Jon Stewart to Join Over One
     Hundred 9/11 First Responders on Sept. 16th As They Walk the Halls of
     Congress Yet Again to Lobby for Continuation oft 9/11 Health Care &
     Compensation Programs They Desperately Need and Deserve," September 8,
     2015, https://www.renew911health.org/press-statement/mr-stewart-goes-to
     -washington-citizens-for-the-extension-of-the-james-zadroga-act-9-11
     -responder-advocate-john-feal-announce-jon-stewart-to-join-over-one-hundred
     -9-11-first-responders-on-s/.

221 Peter Haskell, "Those Sickened After 9/11 Attacks May Be Eligible for
     Free Health Care, Compensation," WCBS 880, September 16, 2019,
     https://wcbs880.radio.com/articles/news/those-sickened-after-911-eligible
     -health care.

222 "Program Statistics," World Trade Center Health Program, CDC, August 13,
     2019, https://www.cdc.gov/wtc/ataglance.html#memberGender.

223 Cameron Joseph and Larry McShane, "Zadroga Act Reauthorization Finally
     Passes Through Congress; Health Care Program Extended 75 Years for 9/11
     First Responders," New York Daily News, December 19, 2015,
     https://www.nydailynews.com/news/politics/zadroga-act-reauthorization
     -finally-passes-congress-article-1.2470110.

224 Ibid.

225 "Program Laws," World Trade Center Health Program, CDC, December 30,
     2019, https://www.cdc.gov/wtc/laws.html.

226 *Program Inventories: Overall Enrollment* (New York: World Trade Center
     Health, 2015), https://www.cdc.gov/wtc/pdfs/statistics/cdata-q1-fy2015-P.pdf.

227 Michele Lent Hirsch, *Invisible: How Young Women with Serious Health Issues
     Navigate Work, Relationships, and the Pressure to Seem Just Fine* (New York:
     Penguin Random House, 2018).

228 Carl Campanile, "Cancer Cluster at Top NYC High School Near Ground Zero,
     Grad Says," *New York Post*, November 9, 2017, https://nypost.com/
     2017/11/09/cancer-cluster-at-high-school-near-ground-zero/.

229 Bob Hennelly, "The Wound That Won't Heal," *City & State New York*, September 10, 2019, https://www.cityandstateny.com/articles/politics/new-york-city/911-the-wound-that-wont-heal.html.

230 Department of Justice, "James Zadroga Health and Compensation Act of 2010 Final Rule," *Federal Register* 76, No. 169 (October 31, 2011): 54112, https://www.federalregister.gov/d/2011-22295/p-24.

231 "Suit Challenging ACA Legally Suspect But Threatens Loss of Coverage for Tens of Millions," Center on Budget and Policy Priorities, November 3, 2020 https://www.cbpp.org/research/health/suit-challenging-aca-legally-suspect-but-threatens-loss-of-coverage-for-tens-of.

232 Karen Pollitz, "Pre-existing Conditions: What Are They and How Many People Have Them?" Kaiser Family Foundation, October 1, 2020, https://www.kff.org/policy-watch/pre-existing-conditions-what-are-they-and-how-many-people-have-them/.

233 Josh Bivens and Ben Zipperer, "Health Insurance and the COVID-19 Shock," Economic Policy Institute, August 26, 2020, https://www.epi.org/publication/health-insurance-and-the-covid-19-shock/.

234 "Health Insurance Coverage of the Total Population," State Health Facts, Kaiser Family Foundation, 2019 https://www.kff.org/other/state-indicator/total-population/?dataView=1&currentTimeframe=0&selectedDistributions=non-group--uninsured&sortModel=%7B%22colId%22:%22Location%22,%22sort%22:%22asc%22%7D.

235 Rachel Black and Aleta Sprague, "The Rise and Reign of the Welfare Queen," New America, September 26, 2016, https://www.newamerica.org/weekly/rise-and-reign-welfare-queen/.

236 Kristen Whitney Daniels, "Poll: Many Americans Still Suspicious of Nations' Welfare System," *National Catholic Reporter*, August 16, 2016, https://www.ncronline.org/blogs/ncr-today/poll-many-americans-still-suspicious-nations-welfare-system.

237 Carrie Healey, "Tania Head: One of the Biggest Frauds in History Pretended to be 9/11 Survivor," AOL, September 10, 2016, https://www.aol.com/article/news/2016/09/10/tania-head-fake-survivor-september-11/21467377/.

238 "Section 7: Information for Individuals with Attorneys," September 11 Victim Compensation Fund, accessed March 25, 2021, https://www.vcf.gov/policy/information-individuals-attorneys.

239 David Goguen, "Lawyers' Fees in Your Personal Injury Case," All Law (blog), https://www.alllaw.com/articles/nolo/personal-injury/lawyers-fees.html.

240 U.S. Congress, House, Committee on The Judiciary Constitution, Civil Rights and Civil Liberties Subcommittee, *The Need to Reauthorize the September 11th Victim Compensation Fund*, 116th Cong., 1st sess, 2019, https://www.justice.gov/opa/speech/september-11th-victim-compensation -fund-special-master-rupa-bhattacharyya-testifies-us.

241 Ibid.

242 Trish Turner, "Sen Tom Coburn Outlines 'Concerns' with 9/11 Health Bill," Fox News, Dec 21, 2010, https://www.foxnews.com/politics/ sen-tom-coburn-outlines-concerns-with-9-11-health-bill.

243 U.S. Department of Justice, "September 11th Victim Compensation Fund, FU 2021 Budget & Performance Plan," February 2020, 8 https://www.justice.gov/ doj/page/file/1246536/download.

244 U.S. Department of Justice, "September 11th Victim Compensation Fund, FU 2021 Budget & Performance Plan," February 2020, 3.

245 Department of Justice, "September 11 Victim Compensation Fund: Compensation of Claims," *Federal Register* 83, no. 182, (October 3, 2018): 49946, https://www.vcf.gov/sites/vcf/files/resources/ VCFNoticeofInquiry201821490.pdf.

246 September 11th Victim Compensation Fund, "Policies and Procedures," December 2019, 16, https://www.vcf.gov/sites/vcf/files/resources/VCFPolicy. pdf.

247 U.S. Congress, House, Committee on the Judiciary Constitution, Civil Rights and Civil Liberties Subcommittee, *The Need to Reauthorize the September 11th Victim Compensation Fund*, 116th Cong., 1st sess, 2019, https://www.justice.gov/opa/speech/september-11th-victim-compensation -fund-special-master-rupa-bhattacharyya-testifies-us.

248 Ibid.

249 "About the Victim Compensation Fund," September 11th Victim Compensation Fund, accessed March 25, 2021, https://www.vcf.gov/about.

250 *Annual Report 2019* (Washington, DC: September 11th Victim Compensation Fund), 17, https://www.vcf.gov/sites/vcf/files/media/document/2020-03/ VCFStatusReportFeb2020.pdf.

251 *Policy and Procedures* (Washington, DC: September 11th Victim Compensation Fund, 2019), 35, sec. 2.1, https://www.vcf.gov/sites/vcf/files/resources/ VCFPolicy.pdf.

252 Neil Bhutta, Andrew C. Chang, Lisa J. Dettling, and Joanne W. Hsu (2020). "Disparities in Wealth by Race and Ethnicity in the 2019 Survey of Consumer Finances," *FEDS Notes*. Washington: Board of Governors of the Federal Reserve System, September 28, 2020, https://doi.org/10.17016/2380-7172.2797.

253 Renee Morand, "It's 2021 and Women Still Make 82 Cents for Every Dollar Earned by a Man," NBC News, March 23, 2021, https://www.nbcnews.com/ know-your-value/feature/ it-s-2021-women-still-make-82-cents-every-dollar-ncna1261755.

254 Emily Moss et al, "The Black-White Wealth Gap Left Black Households More Vulnerable," Brookings Institute, December 8, 2020, https://www.brookings.edu/ blog/up-front/2020/12/08/the-black-white-wealth-gap-left-black-households -more-vulnerable/.

255 Habor Compliance, "Entity Formation Fees by State," https://www.harborcompliance.com/information/entity-formation-fees.

256 Soo Youn, "40% of Americans Don't Have $400 in the Bank for Emergency Expenses: Federal Reserve," ABC, March 24, 2019, https://abcnews.go.com/ US/10-americans-struggle-cover-400-emergency-expense-federal/ story?id=63253846.

257 "Jon Stewart Urges Congress to Fund 9/11 Program" *The Washington Post*, February 25, 2019, https://www.washingtonpost.com/video/national/ jon-stewart-urges-congress-to-fund-911-program/2019/02/25/b578148f -8239-4111-9a11-8a1c3c2c5878_video.html.

258 Ibid.

259 Ibid.

260 Ibid.

261 Sen. Kirsten Gillibrand, "Live Video," Facebook, February 26, 2019, https://www.facebook.com/SenKirstenGillibrand/videos/ 2002490563379423/?v=2002490563379423.

262 Ibid.

263 Ibid.

264 Kristen Lombardi, "While Schumer Slept," *The Village Voice*, February 13, 2007, https://www.villagevoice.com/2007/02/13/while-schumer-slept/.

265 Ibid.

266 Ibid.

267 Ibid.

268 Ibid.

269 Ibid.

270 Jason Duane Hahn, "9/11 First Responder Lou Alvarez Has 69th Round of Chemo after Testimony with Jon Stewart," *People*, June 18, 2019, https://people.com/human-interest/911-first-responder-luis-alvarez-69-rounds -chemo-jon-stewart-testimony/.

271 Jacqueline Modine, MD, *Written Testimony*, prepared for the Committee on the Judiciary, Subcommittee on the Constitution, Civil Rights, and Civil Liberties, June 11, 2019, https://www.congress.gov/116/meeting/house/109609/ witnesses/HHRG-116-JU10-Wstate-MolineJ-20190611.pdf.

272 "September 11 Victim Compensation Fund Reauthorization," C-SPAN video, 2:36:54. June 12, 2019. https://www.c-span.org/video/?461603-1/ jon-stewart-advocates-testify-911-victims-compensation-fund-hearing

273 Ibid.

274 Ibid.

275 Ibid.

276 Richard Alles, "The Forgotten Victims of Sept. 11: Survivors, Not Responders, Also Need Health Help," *New York Daily News*, November 22, 2019, https://www.nydailynews.com/opinion/ny-oped-the-forgotten-victims-of -sept-11-20191122-yx54reeujfclziubfg542bkldu-story.html.

277 Ibid.

278 Ibid.

279 House Judiciary Committee, "Testimony of Anesta St. Rose Henry, Widow of Candidus Henry, Local 79," September 11 Victim Compensation Fund Reauthorization, June 12, 2019, https://docs.house.gov/meetings/JU/ JU10/20190611/109609/HHRG-116-JU10-Wstate-HenryA-20190611.pdf.

280 "September 11 Victim Compensation Fund Reauthorization," C-SPAN video, 2:36:54. June 12, 2019, https://www.c-span.org/video/?461603-1/ jon-stewart-advocates-testify-911-victims-compensation-fund-hearing.

281 Ibid.

282 Ibid.

283 Ibid.

284 Ibid.

285 Ibid.

286 Ibid.

287 Ibid.

288 Ibid.

289 Ibid.

290 Ibid.

291 Author's personal video of the speech.

292 Ibid.

293 Nikki Graf, "A Majority of U.S. Teens Fear a Shooting Could Happen at Their School, and Most Parents Share the Concern," Pew Research Center (blog), April 18, 2018, https://www.pewresearch.org/fact-tank/2018/04/18/a-majority-of-u-s-teens-fear-a-shooting-could-happen-at-their-school-and-most-parents-share-their-concern/.

294 John Biers, "Doubts About Safety of Flint's Water 6 years After Crisis," Phys.org, October 29, 2020, https://phys.org/news/2020-10-safety-flint-years-crisis.html.

295 Daniel Cusick, "Today's Floods Occur Along 'A Very Different' Mississippi River," *Scientific American*, May 13, 2019, https://www.scientificamerican.com/article/todays-floods-occur-along-a-very-different-mississippi-river/; Christopher Ingraham, "Houston Is Experiencing Its Third 500 Year Flood in 3 years. How Is That Possible?" *The Washington Post*, August 29, 2017, https://www.washingtonpost.com/news/wonk/wp/2017/08/29/houston-isexperiencing-its-third-500-year-flood-in-3-years-how-is-that-possible/.

296 Dani Anguiano, "California's Wildfire Hell: How 2020 Became the State's Worst Ever Fire Season," *The Guardian*, December 30, 2020, https://www.theguardian.com/us-news/2020/dec/30/california-wildfires-north-complex-record.

297   Lesley McClurg, "Pandemic Takes Toll on Children's Mental Health," Weekend
       Edition Saturday, NPR, November 28, 2020, https://www.npr.
       org/2020/11/28/938460892/pandemic-takes-toll-on-childrens-mental-health.

298   "Our Story: Not One More," March for Our Lives, accessed March 25, 2021,
       https://marchforourlives.com/mission-story/.

299   Gina Martinez, "GoFundMe CEO: One-Third of Site's Donations Are to Cover
       Medical Costs," *Time*, January 30, 2019, https://time.com/5516037/
       gofundme-medical-bills-one-third-ceo/.

300   Nele Gielen et al., "Prevalence of Post-Traumatic Stress Disorder among Patients
       with Substance Use Disorder: It Is Higher than Clinicians Think It Is," *European
       Journal of Psychotraumatology* 3 (August 2012): https://www.ncbi.nlm.nih.gov/
       pmc/articles/PMC3415609/; D. Ganz and L. Sher, "Suicidal Behavior in
       Adolescents with Post-Traumatic Stress Disorder," *Minerva pediatrica* 62, 4
       (2010): 363–70, https://pubmed. ncbi.nlm.nih.gov/20940670/.

301   Dianne Gallagher et al., "How Parkland Students Feel about Their New
       Mandatory Clear Backpacks," CNN, April 2, 2018, https://www.cnn.
       com/2018/04/02/us/marjory-stoneman-douglas-clear-backpacks/index.html.

302   Travis M. Andrews, "Flint Residents Too Scared of the Water to Wash.
       That's Making Them Sick," *The Washington Post*, October 4, 2010, https://
       www.washingtonpost.com/news/morning-mix/wp/2016/10/04/flint-residents
       -too-scared-of-the-water-to-wash-its-making-them-sick/;
       Jason Kurtis, "Flint Family of 7 Forced to Cook, Bathe with Bottled Water,"
       ABC, January 28, 2016 https://abc7ny.com/news/flint-family-of-7
       -forced-to-cook-bathe-with-bottled-water/1177652/.

303   Robert H. Pietrzak, et al., "Physical Health Conditions Associated with
       Posttraumatic Stress Disorder in U.S. Older Adults: Results from Wave 2 of the
       National Epidemiologic Survey on Alcohol and Related Conditions," *Journal of
       the American Geriatrics Society* 2, vol. 60 (January 27, 2012): 296–303,
       https://www.ncbi.nlm.nih.gov/pmc/articles/PMC3288257/.

304   Charles R. Marmar et al., "Course of Posttraumatic Stress Disorder 40 Years
       After the Vietnam War: Findings from the National Vietnam Veterans
       Longitudinal Study," *JAMA Psychiatry* 72, 9 (September, 2015): 875–881,
       doi:10.1001/jamapsychiatry.2015.0803, https://jamanetwork.com/journals/
       jamapsychiatry/fullarticle/2398184.

305 Karen Davis et al., "Mirror, Mirror 2017: International Comparison Reflects Flaws and Opportunities for Better U.S. Health Care," *The Commonwealth Fund* (2017), https://www.commonwealthfund.org/publications/fund-reports/2017/jul/mirror-mirror-2017-international-comparison-reflects-flaws-and.

306 Lila Nordstrom, "The Dust That Hasn't Settled," *The Guardian*, September 11, 2008, https://www.theguardian.com/commentisfree/cifamerica/2008/sep/11/uselections2008.september11.

307 Centers for Disease Control and Prevention, *WTC Health Program Member Handbook* 3, (July 2020): 1–2, https://www.cdc.gov/wtc/pdfs/handbook/WTCHP_MemberHandbook_2020_EN-P.pdf.

308 Chelsea Parsons et al, "America's Youth Under Fire" (blog), Center for American Progress, May 4, 2018, https://www.americanprogress.org/issues/guns-crime/reports/2018/05/04/450343/americas-youth-fire/.

309 Willem Roper, "Black Americans 2.5x More Likely than Whites to Be Killed by Police," Statista, June 2, 2020, https://www.statista.com/chart/21872/map-of-police-violence-against-black-americans/.

310 Centers for Disease Control and Prevention, "Facts About the WTC Health Program: Overall Enrollment in the WTC Health Program," September 30, 2020, https://www.cdc.gov/wtc/ataglance.html#enrollmentWTC.

311 Eileen Reynolds, "On 9/11 Women Were Heroes Too" (blog), NYU, September 9, 2016, https://www.nyu.edu/about/news-publications/news/2016/september/fdny-captain-brenda-berkman-on-9-11.html.

312 Bob Hennelly, "CMS Unions Protest Double Standard on 9/11 Disability Grants," *Chief Leader*, October 6, 2017, https://thechiefleader.com/news/news_of_the_week/ems-unions-protest-double-standard-on-disability-grants/article_e627a702-9e16-11e7-a4ba-5b0515908f82.html.

313 Ibid.

314 Sarah Jones and Emily Atkins, "Rural America's Drinking Water Crisis," *The New Republic*, February 12, 2018, https://newrepublic.com/article/147011/rural-americas-drinking-water-crisis.

315 Katie Sanders, "Steinem: More Women Killed by Partners since 9/11 than Deaths from Attacks, Ensuing Wars," Politifact (blog), October 7, 2014, https://www.politifact.com/factchecks/2014/oct/07/gloria-steinem/steinem-more-women-killed-partners-911-deaths-atta/.

316 Tiffany N. Ford et al., "Race Gaps in COVID-19 Deaths Are Even Bigger than They Appear," Brookings, June 16, 2020, https://www.brookings.edu/blog/ up-front/2020/06/16/race-gaps-in-covid-19-deaths-are-even-bigger -than-they-appear/.

317 Frances Robles, "Official Toll in Puerto Rico: 64. Actual Deaths May Be 1,052," *The New York Times*, December 9, 2017, https://www.nytimes.com/ interactive/2017/12/08/us/puerto-rico-hurricane-maria-death-toll.html.

318 Adrian Florido, "2 Years After Hurricane Maria Hit Puerto Rico, The Exact Death Toll Remains Unknown," NPR, September 24, 2019, https://www.npr. org/2019/09/24/763958799/2-years-after-hurricane-maria-hit-puerto-rico -the-exact-death-toll-remains-unkno.

319 Centers for Disease Control and Prevention, *WTC Health Program Member Handbook*.

ACKNOWLEDGMENTS

I often refer to myself and my parents as "chaos people." Our little trio is almost always up to shenanigans, and usually, those shenanigans are political. My mom and dad, Carla and Andy, trained me in the art of advocacy from a young age, always modeling the importance of being a good citizen, a principled advocate, and, sometimes, a pain in the ass. It is thanks to their example that I knew where to start in advocating for my classmates, and they've provided moral, physical, financial, and every other conceivable kind of support along the way.

Getting health services for the 9/11 community was a massive group project, and I continue to rely heavily on the support and expertise of many other advocates. Huge thanks are due to 9/11 Environmental Action, especially Kimberly Flynn, Mary Perillo, Barbara Reich, and Rachel Lidov, who have helped fund, support, and bolster my work advocating for and reaching out to young adult survivors for many years. The Stuyvesant Parents' Association and the parents and teachers of Concerned Stuyvesant Community laid the groundwork for my involvement and kept the receipts we'd later need to make our case. Advocates from NYCOSH, Community Board 1, Beyond Ground Zero, Citizens for the Extension of the James Zadroga Act, many downtown unions, and members of the community at large played critical roles in highlighting the need for 9/11 health services in the downtown community, as did many of the WTCHP doctors, administrators, and public officials who have worked to make these services available to and accessible for survivors. Joan Reibman, Rupa Bhattacharyya, Jackie Moline, Dr. John Howard and the staff at NIOSH, and the NYC Department of Health's WTC Health Registry deserve thanks, as does Michael Barasch for finally explaining the VCF to me in idiot-proof language, then making sure I was able to advocate for it at every event, lobbying day, and media appearance leading up to the 2019 renewal.

Beyond the survivor community, massive thanks of course are due to John Feal and the entire FealGood team for walking the halls of Congress with such frequency (and panache) and for inviting me along for the ride. (I'm still waiting for my FealGood polo, though!) To Ben Chevat for pouring so much of his life and expertise into this bill and this cause, to Jon Stewart for using his time, platform, and way with words to demand action on every Zadroga iteration, to the three namesakes of 2019's legislation: Det. Louis Alvarez, Ray Pfeifer, and James Zadroga, who used their last days to make the case that we deserved care, and to our wonderful advocates in Congress, who fought hard to make the WTC Health Program and VCF happen: Reps. Carolyn Maloney, Jerrold Nadler, the "relentless" Sen. Kirsten Gillibrand, and Secretary (and former NY Senator) Hillary Clinton, as well as their dedicated staffers, many of whom I now consider friends.

Speaking of friends, I made the best ones possible at Stuyvesant. Indrina Kanth was my first (and second) reader. Her early feedback and insights were crucial. Kara Benson (I know, technically we didn't meet at Stuy) has been my cheerleader, my coach, and my perennial DC host throughout the lobbying fun. She's never turned me away even though I frequently announce I'm coming at the last minute and eat all of her snacks. Thomas Kunjappu, Carlos Williams, Ryan Muir, Michael Vogel, Ben Magarik, Aarti Surti, Anna Cummings, John Fu, Michele Hirsch, and many others have provided crucial support to StuyHealth's advocacy and outreach work. The Antiguan Eight, Annie Thoms, Tania Strauss, and Nivi Pinnamaneni have offered information, support, cheerleading, and feedback in the course of this book's writing. A few non-Stuy friends offered my first window into what the rest of the world might see reflected in this story. Thanks to Brent Thornburg, Kat Calvin, and Sascha Meisel for reading through those early typo-infused pages and, while all that was going on, helping me ride out the pandemic with my sense of humor intact.

And finally, a massive thanks to the entire team at Apollo, especially Margaret Kaplan, who first contacted me about this project back in mid-2019 and believed me when I said that there was a bigger story to tell about 9/11 than the one most people had heard.

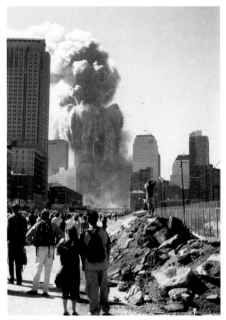

The North Tower falling, with Stuyvesant in the foreground, as evacuees watch. This image was used as the cover of *The Spectator*'s special 9/11 Commemorative Issue, created under editor in chief Jeff Orlowski and faculty advisor Holly Ojalvo.

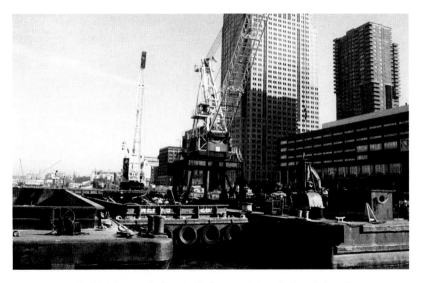

The debris barge, parked just outside Stuyvesant's doors, in the early days of the 9/11 cleanup. Trucks dumped debris there day and night.

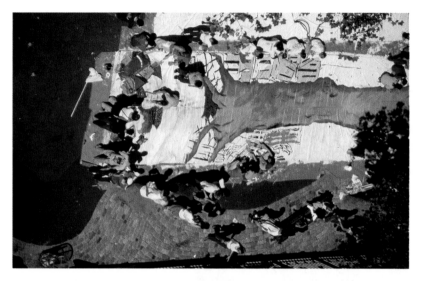

The mural project, organized by a Stuyvesant parent, which drew
Stuyvesant students together in the week after the attacks.

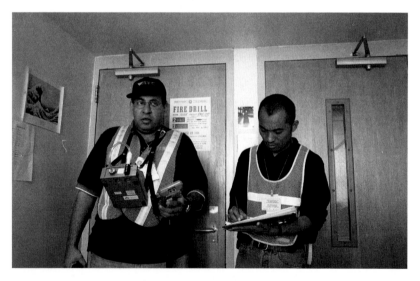

The air quality monitors at Stuyvesant, who would wander
in and out of classrooms taking air readings.

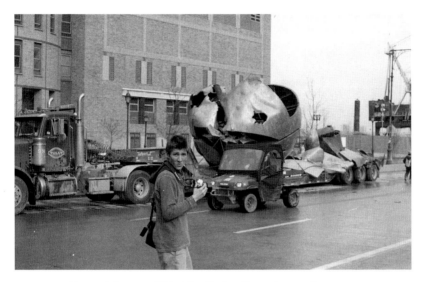

The mangled remains of "The Sphere" by Fritz Koenig, the statue that once sat between the Twin Towers, parked in front of Stuyvesant in early 2002. The remains of the statue were returned to the World Trade Center site in 2017.

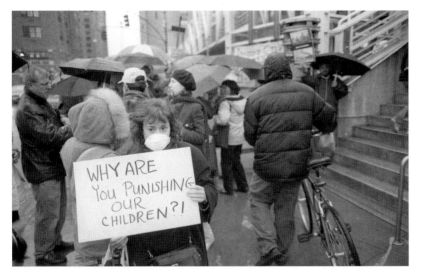

Parents from Stuyvesant and other local schools march outside Stuyvesant in 2002 to protest the decision to return students to the area before it was safe.

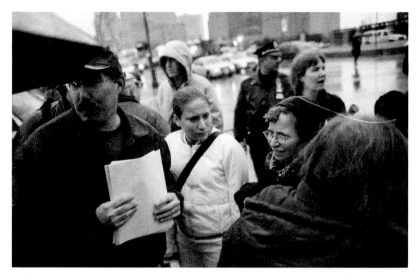

My mother and I at an air quality protest outside Stuyvesant in 2002.

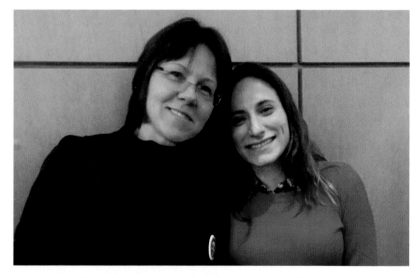

Reuniting with Anetta Luczak, the teacher I evacuated with on 9/11, at an outreach event in 2018. It was the first time we'd seen each other since 2002.

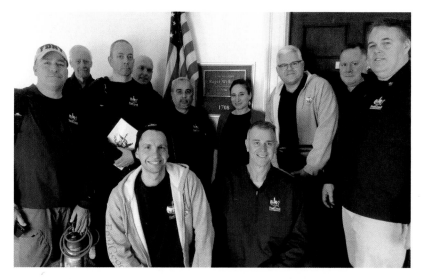

Lobbying on Capitol Hill to extend the Victim Compensation Fund in 2019 along with first responders and advocates from the FealGood Foundation.

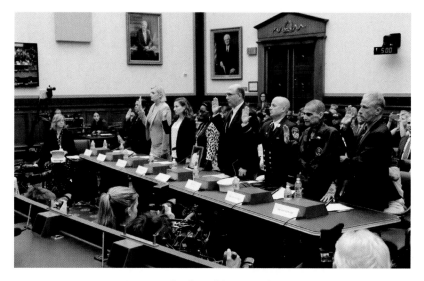

Being sworn in to testify in front of the House Judiciary Committee along with Jon Stewart, Det. Lou Alverez, and others.

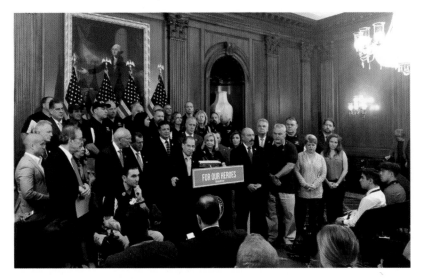

Standing in the huddle with Speaker Nancy Pelosi, House members, Det. Alvarez's family, and FealGood Foundation advocates just ahead of the House of Representative's July 12, 2019 vote on the Victim Compensation Fund.

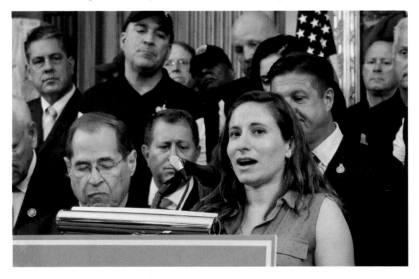

Speaking at a House press conference on July 12, 2019, just before the House vote on the VCF extension.

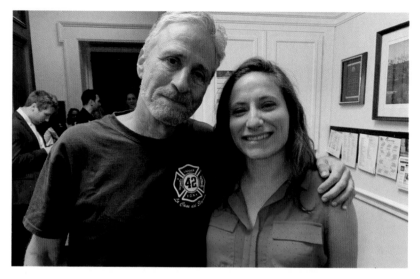

Waiting in Rep. Carolyn B. Maloney's office with Jon Stewart for the House's vote on July 12, 2019.

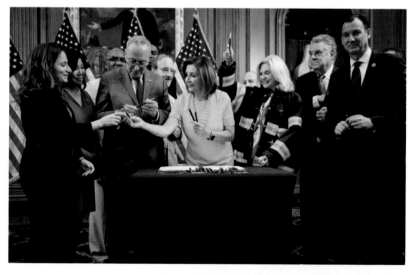

Speaker Nancy Pelosi handing out the pens used to sign Never Forget The Heroes: James Zadroga, Ray Pfeifer, and Luis Alvarez Permanent Authorization of the September 11th Victim Compensation Fund in 2019.

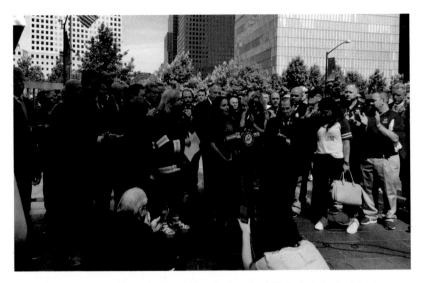

Speaking at a press conference in July 2019 alongside Reps. Jerrold Nadler and Carolyn B. Maloney and first responder advocates, encouraging the Senate to vote on the VCF extension.

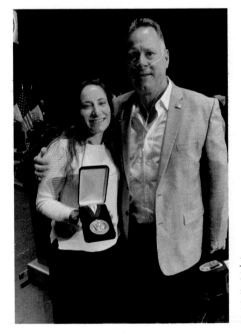

Just after being awarded the Bronze Medallion by the New York City mayor for my role in the Victim Compensation Fund renewal effort alongside my friend Rich Roeill, a 9/11 first responder.